AF765536

WORLD HEALTH ORGANIZATION
EUROPE

Policies and practices for mental health in Europe

- meeting the challenges

Contents

10. Opportunities for the empowerment and representation of service users and carers 143

11. Human rights and mental health 157

12. Information and research on mental health 171

13. Conclusion 179

Annexes 186

Tables and figures

Foreword

I remember with pride the Mental Health Declaration for Europe being signed in Helsinki in 2005 and the strong commitment by governments to address the daunting challenges facing mental health in Europe. Since then, the European Member States have been very active in developing policies and programmes, in many instances in partnership with the WHO Regional Office for Europe. What has been lacking so far, however, has been information and knowledge about the comparative state and progress of mental health and mental health services across the European Region. Such knowledge is important, since it informs about areas in which action could be beneficial, but it also offers examples of excellence that could assist other countries in their development.

I am therefore delighted to present this report on the state of mental health policies and programmes in Europe, co-funded by the European Commission. It is the first report of its kind, offering a wide overview of activities in areas such as mental health promotion, mental disorder prevention, preventing stigma, service provision, human rights and empowerment of service users and families and carers. We hope that this report will be of value to countries, agencies and experts, offering information about mental health activities in many European countries.

A few insights emerge strongly. First, the diversity of the European Region is very apparent. Every table and figure in this report shows variation, and nearly always with a gradient pointing in the same direction. This is obviously related to economies, investment and stages of development, and it calls for solidarity around the Region. Countries complement each other, and we can learn from each other, as demonstrated by the many pilot programmes in existence throughout the Region.

The second message is the growing implementation of community-based mental health services. This report mentions the word "convergence". It is positive that countries have taken to their hearts the vision and evidence supporting deinstitutionalization and establishing services close to where people live. Undeniably, there is still a long way to go, as illustrated by some of the examples of poor institutional practices in this report, but countries now agree that these are no longer acceptable and are introducing alternatives.

An exciting development is the growing involvement of service users and carers in planning services and inspecting mental health facilities. The reluctance to accept this as standard good practice has always surprised me. Everyone seems to agree that the best people to ask for an opinion about products such as radios or software are the people using them. The most successful firms develop products in close partnership with their consumers. This approach must be equally valid in health care. The essence of empowering service users is to consider them valid and autonomous partners. We will be working in this area with the greatest commitment.

Great challenges remain, as presented throughout this report. A major one is the lack of reliable indicators and valid information, hampering meaningful comparisons in many areas. This is well recognized and deserves concerted action in partnership between agencies.

Taking all the findings in this report into account, we believe that we have created strong momentum towards shaping progressive mental health programmes that will serve the diverse needs of our people well. The opportunity now is to build on this momentum, and we hope that this report will encourage the Member States to continue the impressive progress achieved so far.

Marc Danzon
WHO Regional Director for Europe

Acknowledgements

Ionela Petrea and Matt Muijen prepared this report.

We would like to thank:
- Jürgen Scheftlein for continuous support and commitment to this project;
- Anja Baumann for writing the chapter on promoting mental health and preventing mental disorders;
- Andrew McCulloch for contributing to the chapters on policy and legislation on mental health and on opportunities for the empowerment and representation of service users and carers;
- Alan Cohen for contributing to the chapter on mental health in primary care;
- Eva Jane Llopis for contributing to the development of the baseline assessment questionnaire;
- Tom Burns for contributing to the glossary attached to the baseline assessment questionnaire;
- Katherine Moloney for contributing to inputting and cross-checking data;
- Yuliya Zinova for translating the baseline assessment questionnaire into Russian;
- Tina Kiaer for coordinating the production of this report;
- Johanna Kehler for overall administrative support to the project; and
- David Breuer for editing the text.

We are particularly grateful to the Gatsby Charitable Foundation for generous financial support over the years to activities that improve the state of mental health care, including the production of this report.

For the names of the contributors from countries, see Annex 1.

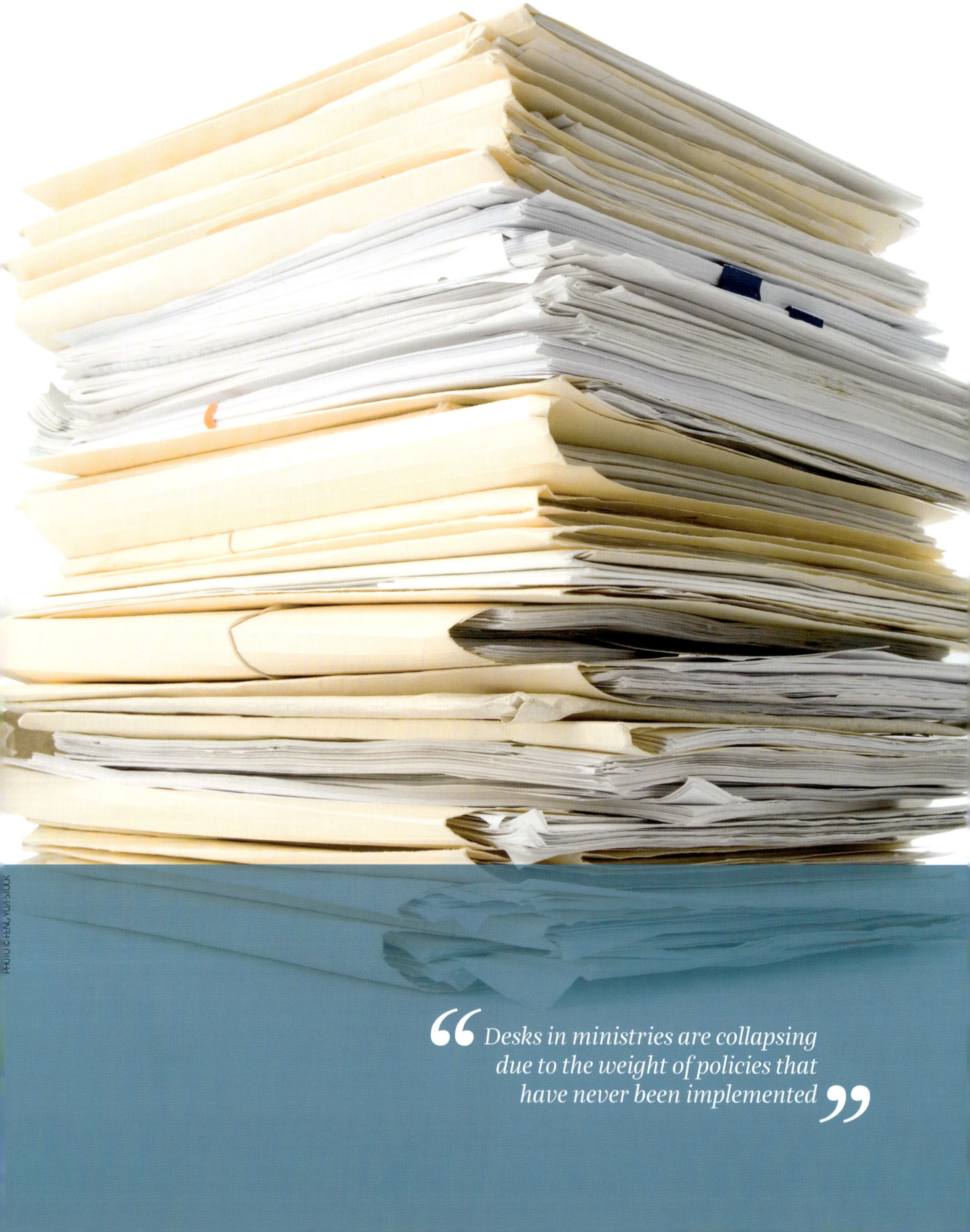

“Desks in ministries are collapsing due to the weight of policies that have never been implemented”

PHOTO © FENG YU/I-STOCK

1. Introduction

Most European countries have recognized mental health as a priority area in recent years. Neuropsychiatric disorders are the second leading cause of disability-adjusted life-years (DALYs) in the WHO European Region, accounting for 19.5% of all DALYs.

According to the most recent available data (2002), neuropsychiatric disorders rank as the first-ranked cause of years lived with disability (YLD) in Europe, accounting for 39.7% of those attributable to all causes. Unipolar depressive disorder alone is responsible for 13.7% of YLD, making it by far the leading cause of chronic conditions in Europe.[1] Alzheimer disease and other forms of dementia are the seventh leading cause of chronic conditions in Europe and account for 3.8% of all YLD. Schizophrenia and bipolar disorders are each responsible for 2.3% of all YLD.

Suicide rates are high in the European Region. The average suicide prevalence rate in Europe is 15.1 per 100 000 population, with the highest rates in the countries in the Commonwealth of Independent States (CIS) (22.7 per 100 000 population) followed by the countries joining the European Union (EU) since 2004 (15.5 per 100 000 population)[2].

In response to this situation, this report is the first ambitious attempt to bring together data on mental health policy and practice from across the European Region of WHO.

In Helsinki, on 17 January 2005, health ministers of the Member States in the WHO European Region endorsed the Mental Health Declaration for Europe: Facing the Challenges, Building Solutions, also referred to as the Helsinki Declaration (Annex 2). In this Declaration, ministers responsible for health committed themselves, "subject to national constitutional structures and responsibilities, to recognizing the need for comprehensive evidence-based mental health policies and to considering ways and means of developing, implementing and reinforcing such policies in our countries."

The Declaration and the Mental Health Action Plan for Europe defined the scope of mental health policy and practice (Box 1.1) and proposed a series of actions in 12 interrelated and interdependent areas to create a comprehensive mental health system. Countries accepted responsibility to support the implementation of measures, and the WHO Regional Office for Europe was requested to take the necessary steps to fully support the development and implementation of mental health policy.

Box 1.1. Scope of mental health policy and practice

- Promoting mental well-being
- Tackling stigma, discrimination and social exclusion
- Preventing mental health problems
- Providing care for people with mental health problems and providing comprehensive and effective services and interventions, offering service users and carers[a] involvement and choice
- Rehabilitating and including into society the people who have experienced serious mental health problems

[a] This publication uses the term "carer" to describe a family member, friend or other informal caregiver.

The WHO Regional Office for Europe has been mandated to take a range of actions and has been actively pursuing these (see Annex 2). Central to its activities are producing comparative data on the state and progress of mental health and mental health services in Member States, with the aim of dissemination and support to develop and implement best policy and practice. This has proven to be a challenge, since essential information is not always available to meet these objectives, and if information is available, it is not always known whether data are standardized and consistent across Member States, since countries had rarely agreed on definitions.

1 *Global burden of disease estimates.* Geneva, World Health Organization, 2004 (http://www.who.int/healthinfo/bodestimates/en/index.html, accessed 8 May 2008).

2 European Health for All database [online database]. Copenhagen, WHO Regional Office for Europe, 2008 (http://data.euro.who.int/hfadb, accessed 8 May 2008).

In response to this, the WHO Regional Office for Europe developed this project, co-funded by the European Commission, to collect and present baseline data about mental health activities in European countries. Its aim was to produce information about the stage of development of the 12 mental health action areas described in the Declaration and Action Plan and to attempt to determine whether progress has been made towards the 12 milestones across Europe (Box 1.2). The aim of identifying progress has to be interpreted with some caution, since this is a survey, which does not allow for good insight into change over time. The survey offers comparisons of the presence of policies and activities in countries. Nevertheless, if data were to be used for benchmarking or auditing exercises, caution is necessary since the concepts, quality of data, collection methods and the structure and delivery of services vary. This report regularly specifies this. Benchmarking was not the aim of this report, since different indicators are necessary for such purposes, and, as the report concludes, much work is yet required to develop them.

A challenge in its own right was whether this survey could meaningfully be conducted and what the next steps should be. This report is the first stage, a baseline, and it is hoped that it will produce productive discussions and challenges resulting in action that will benefit the recipients of mental health policies and practices.

Box 1.2. Milestones of the Mental Health Action Plan for Europe

Member States are committed, through the Mental Health Declaration for Europe and this Action Plan, to face the challenges by moving towards the following milestones. Between 2005 and 2010 they should:

1. prepare policies and implement activities to counter stigma and discrimination and promote mental well-being, including in healthy schools and workplaces;
2. scrutinize the mental health impact of public policy;
3. include the prevention of mental health problems and suicide in national policies;
4. develop specialist services capable of addressing the specific challenges of the young and older people, and gender-specific issues;
5. prioritize services that target the mental health problems of marginalized and vulnerable groups, including problems of comorbidity, i.e. where mental health problems occur jointly with other problems such as substance misuse or physical illness;
6. develop partnership for intersectoral working and address disincentives that hinder joint working;
7. introduce human resource strategies to build up a sufficient and competent mental health workforce;
8. define a set of indicators on the determinants and epidemiology of mental health and for the design and delivery of services in partnership with other Member States;
9. confirm health funding, regulation and legislation that is equitable and inclusive of mental health;
10. end inhumane and degrading treatment and care and enact human rights and mental health legislation to comply with the standards of United Nations conventions and international legislation;
11. increase the level of social inclusion of people with mental health problems; and
12. ensure representation of users and carers on committees and groups responsible for the planning, delivery, review and inspection of mental health activities.

"There is a striking variation in staff numbers, differences in education and a lack of reliable information available from countries in many areas"

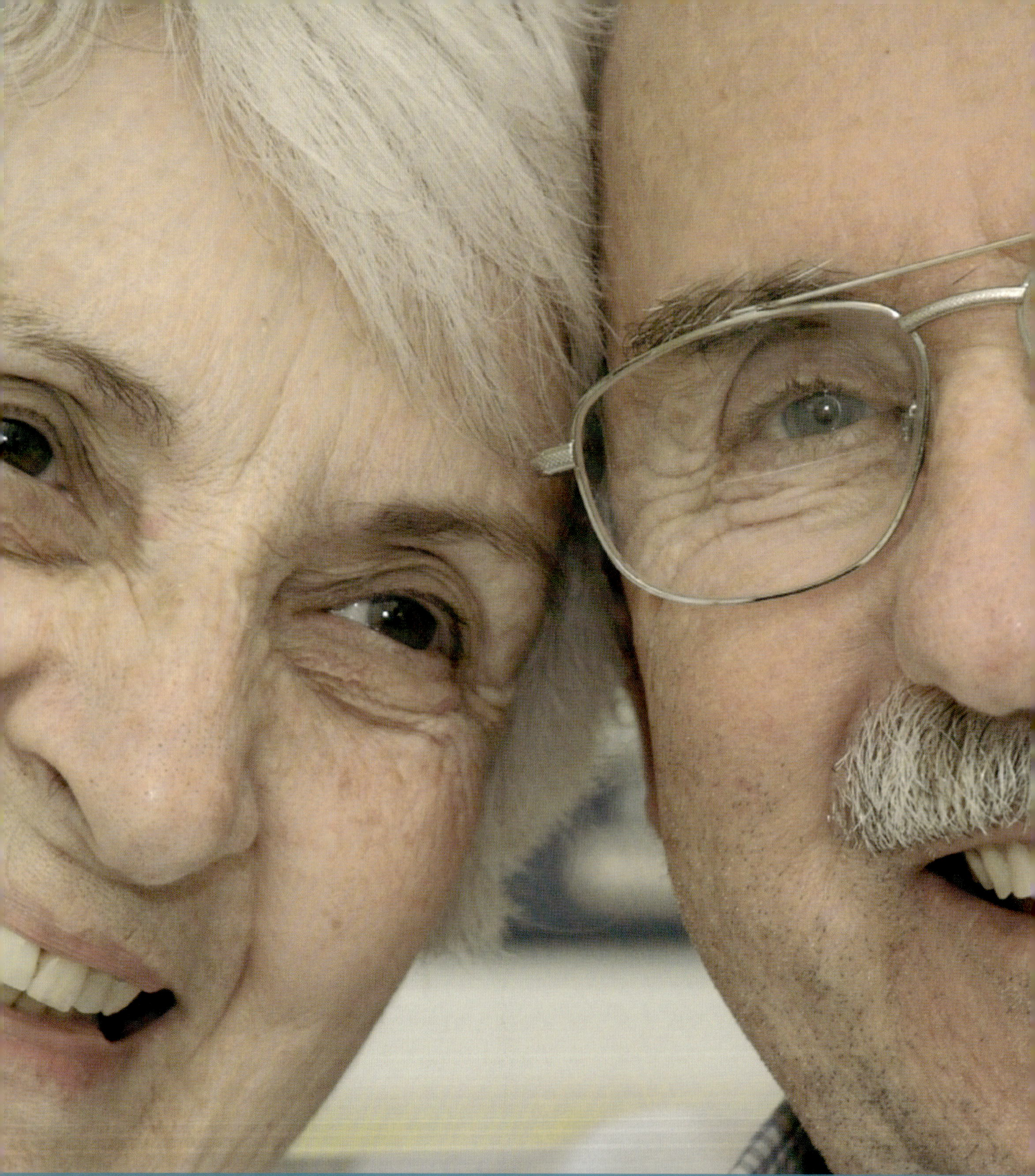

PHOTO © SEAN WARREN/ ISTOCK

"Funding distribution seems to be based on historical allocation or more informal allocation arrangements. Countries could exchange experiences in this field"

2. Methods

The participating countries were requested to complete the baseline assessment questionnaire, an instrument initially designed by the WHO Regional Office for Europe and further developed in consultation with the national counterparts from the participating countries.

Content of the baseline assessment questionnaire

The questionnaire contains 90 questions distributed across the 12 milestones in the Mental Health Action Plan for Europe, introduced by a section focusing on overall mental health policies and legislation. The topics covered are:

- mental health policy and legislation – 7 questions;
- mental health promotion – 9 questions;
- centrality of mental health – 4 questions;
- prevention of mental disorders and suicide – 4 questions;
- mental health services for children and adolescents and older people – 5 questions;
- mental health services for adults – 14 questions:
  - mental health in primary care – 3 questions;
  - specialist mental health services – 11 questions;
- intersectoral partnerships – 5 questions;
- human resources – 12 questions:
  - availability – 5 questions;
  - competencies – 7 questions;
- information and research – 9 questions;
- funding – 7 questions;
- human rights – 6 questions;
- social inclusion – 3 questions; and
- empowerment of users and carers – 5 questions.

A glossary was attached to the questionnaire to facilitate common understanding of the key concepts in the questionnaire. It included 62 definitions that had as its source other WHO documents, specialist papers and books and input from experts (list of sources available from the WHO Regional Office for Europe).

The questionnaire and glossary can be found on the WHO Regional Office web site (http://www.euro.who.int/mentalhealth/ctryinfo/20030829_1).

Development of the questionnaire

Staff members of the WHO Regional Office for Europe prepared the first draft questionnaire and its glossary. Previously developed tools for assessing the mental health systems in countries were checked. In particular, the WHO Assessment Instrument for Mental Health Systems[1] (an instrument primarily intended for assessing mental health systems in low- and middle-income countries) was consulted and contributed several questions in the baseline assessment questionnaire.

The first draft of the baseline assessment questionnaire was sent to four countries (Belgium, Italy, Poland and the United Kingdom (England and Wales)) for pre-testing on 10 October 2006. Feedback was incorporated into the second draft of the questionnaire.

A consultative meeting was organized in Vienna, Austria on 26–27 October 2006 for national counterparts from the countries participating in the project to discuss and review the questionnaire. Discussions focused both on the structure of the questionnaire and its content. Changes made at the meeting included:

- adding the introductory section on mental health policy and legislation;
- modifying several questions and removing others;
- adding new questions (the second draft had 82 questions and the final version contains 90 questions); and
- clarifying the concepts used in the glossary.

The third draft was circulated to all participating countries for review between 8 November 2006 and 15 December 2006.

The questionnaire included a few additional changes. Five countries selected by the national counterparts at the Vienna meeting piloted the questionnaire: Belgium, Denmark, Italy, Romania and United Kingdom (Scotland). This stage lasted from 5 January until 15 March 2007. Feedback from the pilot phase was

1 *WHO Assessment Instrument for Mental Health Systems.* Version 2.2. Geneva, World Health Organization, 2005 (WHO/MSD/MER/05.2; http://www.who.int/mental_health/evidence/AIMS_WHO_2_2.pdf, accessed 8 May 2008).

used to prepare the final baseline assessment questionnaire. It was sent to national counterparts in the participating countries on 22 March 2007.

Languages

The questionnaire was made available to the participating countries in English (online and Word versions) and Russian (the Word version only). However, countries were asked to submit the completed questionnaire in English.

Data collection

Timeline

The completed questionnaires were submitted and the data were collected by the end of 2007.

The data collection process

The health ministries of the participating countries were responsible for completing this questionnaire. Following discussions at the Vienna meeting, it was agreed that a national coordinator would be designated in each country (in some countries 2–3 people shared this task). The people nominated were responsible for planning and supervising the data collection and sending the completed questionnaire to the Mental Health Unit of the WHO Regional Office for Europe.

Data collection was a partnership process in many countries, considering the wide range of subjects covered by the questionnaire and to ensure access to accurate and comprehensive information. The national coordinator would receive and coordinate input from national experts in other institutions and organizations in the country.

Data submission

Countries were offered the option of submitting the questionnaire as an online survey or as a Word document.

The online survey was developed with external information technology assistance. An account was created for each country, and the national focal point was sent the link to this account, with instructions on how to complete the questionnaire online (including how to save data, how to browse through the questionnaire, how to review the answers provided, how to submit the questionnaire and how to review and update data after submission). Further information and support were provided to countries on request. Throughout the process, focal points could contact mental health staff at the WHO Regional Office for Europe for assistance.

Data sources and data cross-checking

This project did not intend nor did it have the capacity to check the validity of the primary sources of the data received, and the data presented in this report therefore reflect the information provided and confirmed by the responsible people in the participating countries.

In the questionnaire, the participating countries were asked to indicate the sources of some of the data provided, such as national sources, expert knowledge and international sources.

The data received were scrutinized and further clarification was requested for inconsistency on data submitted and qualifiers for some findings. Outliers were identified, and the focal points were asked to double-check the respective data.

Further, to ensure the quality of the data in the final report, data received from countries were cross-checked with other secondary sources of data such as the WHO *Mental health atlas 2005*,[2] the WHO *Atlas: nurses in mental health 2007*[3] and the WHO European Health for All database.[4] When discrepancies between data available from different sources were identified, countries were asked to confirm which set of data is correct.

2 *Mental health atlas 2005*. Geneva, World Health Organization, 2005 (http://www.who.int/globalatlas/default.asp, accessed 8 May 2008).

3 *Atlas: nurses in mental health 2007*. Geneva, World Health Organization, 2007 (http://www.who.int/mental_health/evidence/nursing_atlas_2007.pdf, accessed 8 May 2008).

4 WHO European Health for All database [online database]. Copenhagen, WHO Regional Office for Europe, 2008 (http://data.euro.who.int/hfadb, accessed 8 May 2008).

Participating countries

Forty-two countries in the WHO European Region participated in this project:

- all 27 EU countries: Austria, Belgium, Bulgaria, Cyprus, Czech Republic, Denmark, Estonia, Finland, France, Germany, Greece, Hungary, Ireland, Italy, Latvia, Lithuania, Luxembourg, Malta, Netherlands, Poland, Portugal, Romania, Slovakia, Slovenia, Spain, Sweden and the United Kingdom;[5]
- seven countries from south-eastern Europe: Albania, Bosnia and Herzegovina (Federation of Bosnia and Herzegovina and Republika Srpska), Croatia, Montenegro, Serbia, the former Yugoslav Republic of Macedonia and Turkey;
- five CIS countries: Azerbaijan, Georgia, Moldova, Russian Federation and Uzbekistan; and
- Israel, Norway and Switzerland.

This survey aimed to capture the information for the whole country. However, in the cases where such information was not available, such as due to regional differences or incomplete information, countries were asked to specify for each question to which regions or areas it applied.

While some countries with a federal structure provided information combining input from different regions (Austria, Germany and Switzerland), others provided separate sets of data for participating regions.

- Bosnia and Herzegovina: based on the agreement between WHO and the country on technical work, information from the Federation of Bosnia and Herzegovina and Republika Srpska was collected separately, and the data on individual variables are presented individually. However, they are counted as one country. Data on the Bosnia and Herzegovina overall (used in tables that present the findings by groups of countries) reflect combined answers from the Federation of Bosnia and Herzegovina and from Republika Srpska.
- Belgium: the information presented in this report refers mainly to data collected from the Flemish Government, except for data on beds per 100 000 population, admissions to inpatient services and the numbers of mental health personnel, which apply to the national level. Some examples of programmes implemented in the Walloon Region and in Brussels-Capital Region are also provided.
- Spain: Spain has 17 autonomous regions, each with its own independent health system. The data for Spain are based on replies from the five regions that responded to the survey: Castilla y León, Catalonia, Extremadura, Galicia and Murcia. The data presented in figures and tables are presented individually for each region, except for data on the numbers of mental health personnel, which represents the median value for all the regions in Spain (source: Observatorio de Salud Mental de la Asociación Española de Neuropsiquiatría, http://www.observatorio-aen.es/cuestionario-observatorio/index.php). The data on Spain overall (when used in tables) reflect a combined answer for the five regions.
  - If at least one region replied "yes", the reply for Spain is registered as "yes".
  - For questions on the proportion of people who have access to certain interventions, the highest value was selected.
  - If the "yes" answer or the higher value applies only to a minority of the responding regions, these regions are indicated in the text.
- United Kingdom: since data were submitted separately for England and Wales and for Scotland, the data on individual variables are presented individually. However, they are counted as one country. Data on the United Kingdom overall (used in tables that present the findings by groups of countries) reflect combined answers from England and Wales and from Scotland.

5 The EU15 countries comprise Austria, Belgium, Denmark, Finland, France, Germany, Greece, Ireland, Italy, Luxembourg, Netherlands, Portugal, Spain, Sweden and the United Kingdom. The countries joining the EU since 2004 comprise Bulgaria, Cyprus, the Czech Republic, Estonia, Hungary, Latvia, Lithuania, Malta, Poland, Romania, Slovakia and Slovenia.

Data analysis

Recording of the data

For the data analysis, the raw data from the countries that submitted the completed questionnaire online (n = 30) was extracted into an Excel document to minimize errors in data recording. The data from the countries that submitted the completed questionnaire in the Word version (n = 12) were entered into this Excel document, and the data were checked to ensure that the input was correct.

Methods of analysis

Categorical data were analysed using the SPSS-14 package. The main function used was cross-tabulation.

"The most promising area is probably identifying and disseminating good evidence, allowing local agencies to adapt this for local implementation"

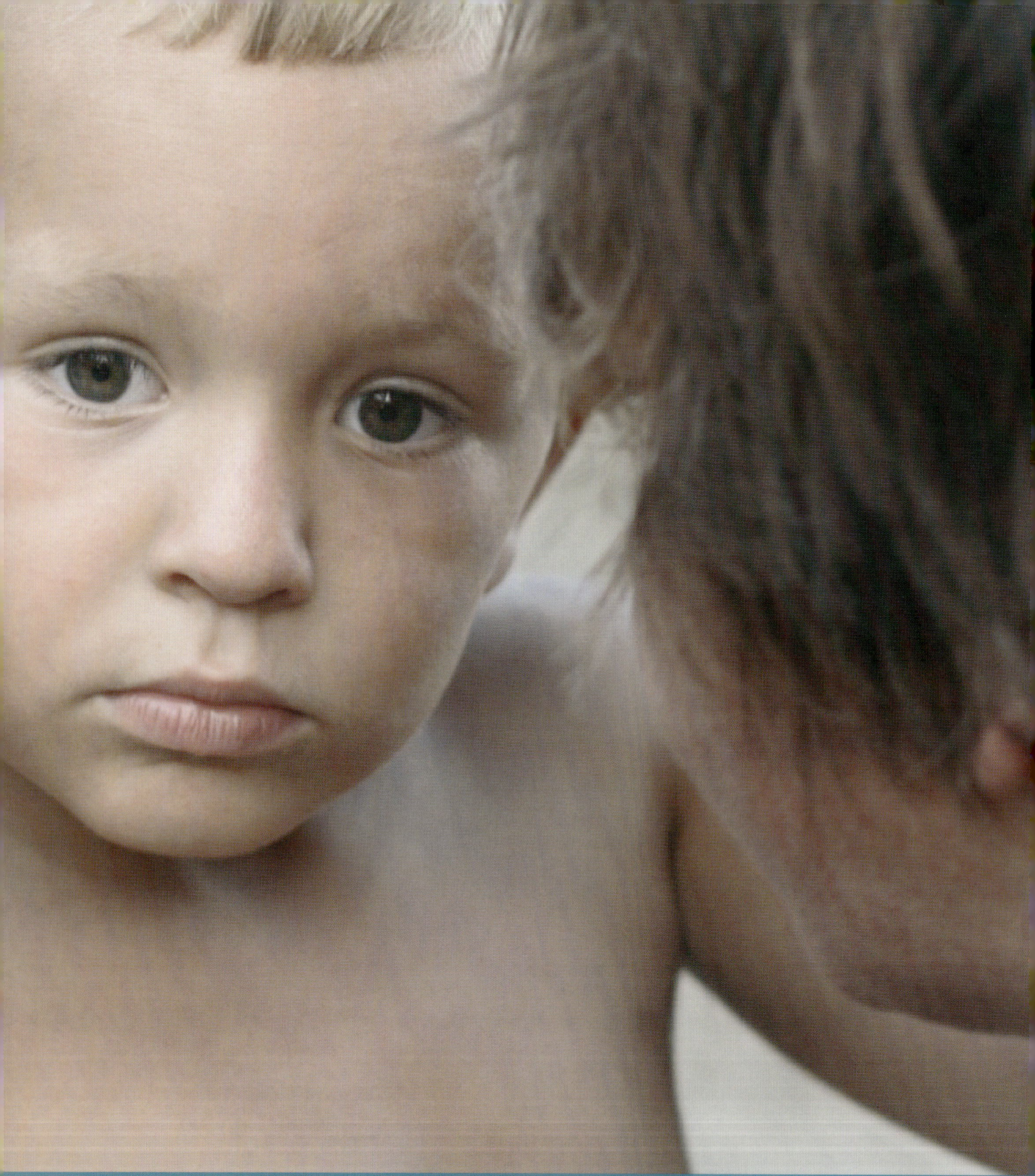

PHOTO © GRIGORY BIBIKOV/ISTOCK

“In much of the eastern part of the Region GPs are actively discouraged, sometimes even by legislation, from becoming involved with mental disorders”

3. Policy and legislation on mental health

Mental health policy and legislation are the foundation on which to develop action and services. Policies are necessary to define the values, direction, responsibilities, structure, functioning and outcomes of services. The Mental Health Declaration for Europe and Mental Health Action Plan for Europe contain much of the content that a mental health policy should cover.

Definitions

For the purposes of this survey, mental health policy has been defined as an organized set of values, principles and objectives aimed at improving mental health and reducing the burden of mental disorder in a population. Such policy is formulated and put into operation in mental health policies, which obtain recognized status following approval by a legal authority, whether a minister, government or parliament.

Approved mental health legislation has been defined as legal provisions related to mental health enacted and implemented by the relevant authorities, typically focusing on such issues as the civil and human rights protection of people with mental disorders, treatment facilities, personnel, professional training and service structure.

Many countries are reducing the numbers of beds and are moving towards closing mental hospitals to replace such institutional forms of care with community-based mental health services. Strategies are therefore especially important to communicate the underlying change in values. Community-based services place great emphasis on people's autonomy and providing care that is based on the needs of the individuals and sensitive to their life experiences and culture. Strategies have to reflect this. Further, introducing community-based services considerably changes the rights, duties and protection of individuals, families, staff and the community. High activity in policy-making and legislation can therefore be predicted in the WHO European Region.

Mental health policy

Countries were asked to indicate whether they have adopted a national mental health policy, either as a separate document or included in overall health policy documents. They were also asked to specify what aspects of mental health policy this policy addresses.

According to WHO guidelines,[1] a comprehensive mental health policy should address the following issues:

- the organization of services: developing community mental health services, downsizing large mental hospitals and developing a mental health component in primary health care;
- the organization of services or initiatives for preventing mental disorders and promoting mental health;
- the quantity and quality of human resources;
- the involvement of users and families and carers;
- advocacy;
- equity of access to mental health services across different groups;
- funding; and
- quality assurance and information systems.

All but 4 of the 42 countries (Azerbaijan, Estonia, Georgia and Moldova) have adopted mental health policies.

The format and content of the mental health policies varies across the European Region: 21 of 42 countries (50%) have produced a mental health policy as a separate document; 6 of 42 countries (14%) have a combination of a specific mental health policy, but other health policies cover some relevant components.

1 *The mental health context* (Mental health policy and service guidance package). Geneva, World Health Organization, 2003 (http://www.who.int/mental_health/resources/en/context.PDF, accessed 8 May 2008).

Table 3.1. Content and components included in approved strategic documents relevant to mental health – strategies, policies or plans in countries

COUNTRY	Organization of services: developing community mental health services	Organization of services: downsizing large mental hospitals	Organization of services: developing a mental health component in primary health care	Organization of services and initiatives for preventing mental disorders	Organization of initiatives for promoting mental health	Quantity and quality of human resources	Involvement of service users, families and carers	Advocacy	Equity of access to mental health services across different groups	Financing	Quality assurance	Information system
Albania	Yes	Yes	Yes	Yes	Yes	Yes	Yes	Yes	No	Yes	No	Yes
Austria	Yes	Yes	Yes	No	No	No	No	No	No	Yes	No	No
Azerbaijan	Not applicable	Not applicable	Not applicable	Not applicable	Not applicable	Not applicable	Not applicable	Not applicable	Not applicable	Not applicable	Not applicable	Not applicable
Belgium	Yes	Yes	Yes	Yes	Yes	Yes	Yes	Yes	Yes	Yes	Yes	Yes
Bosnia and Herzegovina												
Federation of Bosnia and Herzegovina	Yes	Yes	Yes	Yes	Yes	Yes	Yes	Yes	Yes	Yes	Yes	Yes
Republika Srpska	Yes	Yes	Yes	Yes	Yes	Yes	Yes	Yes	Yes	Yes	Yes	Yes
Bulgaria	Yes	Yes	Yes	Yes	Yes	Yes	Yes	Yes	Yes	Yes	Yes	Yes
Croatia	Yes	Yes	Yes	Yes	Yes	Yes	Yes	Yes	Yes	Yes	Yes	Yes
Cyprus	Yes	Yes	Yes	Yes	No	No	No	No	Yes	Yes	No	No
Czech Republic	Yes	Yes	Yes	No	No	Yes	No	No	Yes	No	No	No
Denmark	Yes	Yes	Yes	Yes	Yes	Yes	Yes	Yes	Yes	Yes	Yes	Yes
Estonia	Not applicable	Not applicable	Not applicable	Not applicable	Not applicable	Not applicable	Not applicable	Not applicable	Not applicable	Not applicable	Not applicable	Not applicable
Finland	Yes	No	Yes	Yes	Yes	Yes	Yes	No	No	No	Yes	Yes
France	Yes	Yes	Yes	Yes	Yes	Yes	Yes	Yes	Yes	Yes	Yes	Yes
Georgia	No	No	No	No	Yes	No	No	No	No	No	No	No
Germany	Yes	Yes	Yes	Yes	Yes	Yes	Yes	Yes	Yes	Yes	Yes	Yes
Greece	Yes	Yes	No	Yes	No	No	No	No	Yes	Yes	Yes	Yes
Hungary	Yes	Yes	Yes	Yes	No	No	No	No	No	No	No	No
Ireland	Yes	Yes	Yes	Yes	Yes	Yes	Yes	Yes	Yes	Yes	No	Yes
Israel	Yes	Yes	Yes	No	Information not available	Yes	Yes	Yes	Yes	Yes	Yes	Yes
Italy	Yes	Not applicable	Yes	Yes	Yes	Yes	Yes	No	Yes	Yes	Yes	Yes
Latvia	Yes	No	No	Yes	Yes	No	No	Yes	No	No	Yes	Yes
Lithuania	Yes	Yes	Yes	Yes	Yes	Yes	Yes	Yes	No	Yes	Yes	Yes
Luxembourg	Yes	Yes	Yes	Yes	Yes	Yes	Yes	Yes	Yes	Yes	Yes	Yes
Malta	Yes	Yes	Yes	Yes	Yes	Yes	Yes	Yes	No	Yes	Yes	No
Moldova	Yes	No	Yes	Yes	Yes	Yes	Yes	Yes	Yes	Yes	Yes	Yes
Montenegro	Yes	No	Yes	Yes	Yes	Yes	Yes	Yes	Yes	Yes	Yes	Yes
Netherlands	Yes	Yes	Yes	Yes	Yes	Yes	Yes	Yes	Yes	Yes	Yes	Yes

Yes ■ No ■ Not applicable ■ Information not available

Table 3.1. continued

COUNTRY	Organization of services: developing community mental health services	Organization of services: downsizing large mental hospitals	Organization of services: developing a mental health component in primary health care	Organization of services and initiatives for preventing mental disorders	Organization of initiatives for promoting mental health	Quantity and quality of human resources	Involvement of service users, families and carers	Advocacy	Equity of access to mental health services across different groups	Financing	Quality assurance	Information system
Norway	Yes	Yes	Yes	Yes	Yes	Yes	Yes	Yes	Yes	Yes	Yes	Yes
Poland	Yes	Yes	Yes	Yes	Yes	Yes	Yes	Yes	Yes	Yes	Yes	Yes
Portugal	Yes	Yes	Yes	Yes	Yes	Yes	Yes	Yes	Yes	Yes	Yes	Yes
Romania	Yes	No	Yes	Yes	Yes	Yes	Yes	Yes	Yes	Yes	No	No
Russian Federation	Yes	Yes	Yes	Yes	Yes	Yes	No	No	Yes	Yes	Yes	Information not available
Serbia	Yes	Yes	Yes	Yes	Yes	Yes	Yes	Yes	Yes	Yes	Yes	Yes
Slovakia	Yes	Yes	Yes	Information not available	Information not available	Yes	Information not available	No	Yes	Yes	No	Yes
Slovenia	No	No	Yes	Yes	Yes	Yes	No	No	No	Yes	No	No
Spain	Yes	Yes	Yes	Yes	Yes	No	Yes	Yes	Yes	Yes	Yes	Yes
Castilla y León	Yes	Yes	Yes	Yes	Yes	Yes	Yes	Yes	Yes	Yes	Yes	Yes
Catalonia	Yes	Yes	Yes	Yes	Yes	Yes	Yes	Yes	Yes	Yes	Yes	Yes
Extremadura	Yes	Yes	Yes	Yes	Yes	Yes	Yes	Information not available	Yes	No	Yes	Yes
Galicia	Yes	Yes	Yes	Yes	No	Yes	Yes	No	Yes	Yes	Yes	Yes
Murcia	Yes	Yes	Yes	Yes	Yes	Yes	Yes	Information not available	Yes	Yes	Yes	Yes
Sweden	Yes	Yes	Yes	No	No	No	Yes	Yes	Yes	No	No	No
Switzerland	Yes	Yes	Yes	Yes	Yes	Yes	Yes	Yes	Yes	Yes	Yes	Yes
The former Yugoslav Republic of Macedonia	Yes	Yes	Yes	Yes	Yes	Yes	Yes	Yes	Yes	Yes	Yes	Yes
Turkey	Yes	Yes	Yes	Yes	Yes	Yes	Yes	Yes	Yes	Yes	Yes	Yes
United Kingdom												
England and Wales	Yes	Yes	Yes	Yes	Yes	Yes	Yes	Yes	Yes	Yes	Yes	Yes
Scotland	Yes	Yes	Yes	Yes	Yes	Yes	Yes	Yes	Yes	Yes	Yes	Yes
Uzbekistan	Yes	Yes	Yes	Yes	Yes	Yes	Yes	Yes	Yes	Yes	Information not available	Yes

Yes · No · Not applicable · Information not available

Mental health policies are incorporated into general health policies in 13 of 42 countries (31%). This includes 4 EU15 countries (Austria, Finland, Luxembourg and Sweden) and 5 of the 12 countries that became EU members after 2004 (Cyprus, Hungary, Latvia, Poland and Slovenia). Moldova has covered several mental health policy components in their general health policy.

Most countries cover all these subjects in their mental health policies (Table 3.1). The most frequent component is developing community services (38 of 42 countries, 90%), and the least frequent is quality assurance (28 of 42 countries, 67%).

Downsizing large mental hospitals is on the policy agenda of 87% of the EU15 countries and 67% of the countries that became EU members after 2004 but only 40% of the CIS countries participating in the survey.

Main developments since 2005

More than half the 42 countries report adopting new mental health policies or updating their existing policies since 2005: Austria, Belgium, Bosnia and Herzegovina (Federation of Bosnia and Herzegovina), Bosnia and Herzegovina (Republika Srpska), Bulgaria, Croatia, Cyprus, Denmark, France, Germany, Ireland, Israel, Italy, Lithuania, Norway, Poland, Portugal, Romania, Russian Federation, Serbia, Spain, Switzerland, the former Yugoslav Republic of Macedonia, Turkey and United Kingdom (Scotland) (Table 3.2, Fig. 3.1).

Some CIS countries are currently preparing national mental health policies under the coordination of lead mental health specialists in these countries and with technical assistance from WHO. At this point, about 40% of the CIS countries participating in the survey have a mental health policy document.

Although some countries have developed and updated their overall mental health strategy, other countries have focused on specific areas such as suicide prevention (Belgium), depression and dementia (Germany), alcohol and drug dependence (Poland and Spain (Murcia)) and mental health promotion (Switzerland).

Other developments in policy include establishing national institutes for mental health (Croatia and Romania), designating a Federal Government Commissioner for Patients' Affairs (Germany), establishing or revising advisory boards for mental health (Austria, Italy and Slovakia) and organizing meetings for key stakeholders (Georgia, Germany, Portugal, Switzerland and Uzbekistan).

Mental health legislation

All countries reported that mental health legislation is in place. Of the 42 countries, 20 (47%) have adopted new mental health legislation or updated their legislation since 2005, and 14 (33%) of the countries have legislation in place that is less than 10 years old (Table 3.3 and Fig. 3.2).

Almost seventy per cent of the countries (29 of 42) have dedicated mental health legislation, and 13 (31%) have provisions about mental health as part of general health legislation. Six countries (14%) cover mental health issues by combining specific mental health and general health legislation.

The adoption of mental health legislation has been decentralized in some countries with a federal structure, and legislation can therefore differ between regions.

The scope of mental health legislation varies across countries. WHO guidance on human rights and mental health legislation[2,3] suggests that comprehensive mental health legislation address a range of topics, including:

- access to mental health care and access to care in community settings;
- the legal rights of mental health service users and of family members and other carers;
- competence or capacity issues for people with mental illness;
- guardianship issues for people with mental illness;

2 *WHO resource book on mental health, human rights and legislation.* Geneva, World Health Organization, 2005 (http://www.who.int/mental_health/policy/legislation/policy/en, accessed 8 May 2008).

3 *Mental health legislation and human rights* (Mental health policy and service guidance package). Geneva, World Health Organization, 2003 (http://www.who.int/mental_health/resources/en/Legislation.pdf, accessed 8 May 2008).

Table 3.2. Period in which the latest policy on mental health was adopted in groups of countries

	EU		EU15		New EU countries since 2004		Israel, Norway and Switzerland		South-eastern Europe		CIS		Total	
Time period	No.	%	No.	%	No.	%	No.	%	No.	%	No.	%	No.	%
After 2005	15	56	10	67	5	42	3	100	5	71	1	20	24	57
1999–2004	9	33	4	27	5	42	0	0	2	29	1	20	12	29
Before 1998	2	7	1	7	1	8	0	0	0	0	0	0	2	5
Never	1	4	0	0	1	8	0	0	0	0	3	60	4	10

- mechanisms to oversee involuntary admission;
- procedures and safeguards for voluntary and involuntary treatment;
- mechanisms to monitor involuntary treatment practices;
- accreditation of professionals and of facilities;
- law enforcement and other judicial system issues for people with mental disorders; and
- mechanisms to implement the provisions of mental health legislation.

The mental health legislation in most countries addresses most of the areas raised in the WHO guidance (Table 3.4). Bulgaria, the Czech Republic, Estonia, Finland, Georgia, Greece, Ireland, Lithuania, Montenegro, Portugal, Serbia and the former Yugoslav Republic of Macedonia do not include such a key area as guardianship issues for people with mental illness in mental health legislation. Nevertheless, a survey focusing on specialized mental health policy and legislation cannot determine whether this area is being genuinely ignored or is covered by other legislation related to guardianship in general. The same could apply to mechanisms to monitor involuntary treatment practices, which Azerbaijan, Bulgaria, Estonia, Greece, Serbia, Slovakia and Switzerland do not include in mental health legislation.

The absence of specified legal rights for families and carers is of some concern, since they are often deeply involved in and affected by the treatment of their relatives.

Fig. 3.1. Year in which the latest policy on mental health was adopted in countries

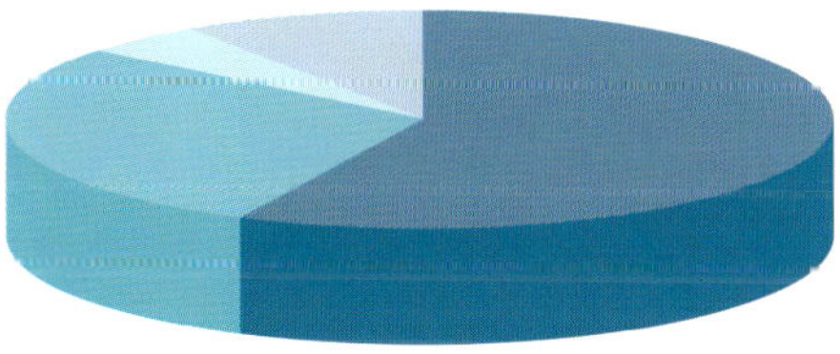

After 2005:
Austria, Belgium, Bosnia and Herzegovina (Federation of Bosnia and Herzegovina and Republika Srpska), Bulgaria, Croatia, Cyprus, Denmark, France, Germany, Ireland, Israel, Italy, Lithuania, Norway, Poland, Portugal, Romania, Russian Federation, Serbia, Spain (Catalonia, Extremadura, Galicia and Murcia), Switzerland, the former Yugoslav Republic of Macedonia, Turkey, United Kingdom (Scotland)

1999–2004:
Albania, Czech Republic, Finland, Greece, Hungary, Latvia, Luxembourg, Montenegro, Netherlands, Slovakia, Slovenia, Spain (Castilla y León), United Kingdom (England and Wales), Uzbekistan

Before 1998:
Malta, Sweden

No policy:
Azerbaijan, Estonia, Georgia, Moldova

Capacity issues, which three of the EU15 countries (20%) do not include in mental health legislation, are often the subject of separate capacity legislation of a complex nature, since its priority groups are people with intellectual disability and dementia. This survey did not cover whether countries have such legislation, which is crucial to the human rights of the most vulnerable people.

Some countries indicate challenges they face in implementing mental health legislation:

- Azerbaijan: the legislation has addressed these issues, but there are no implementation mechanisms and no monitoring of compliance.

Table 3.3. Year in which the latest legislation on mental health was adopted in groups of countries

Time period	EU		EU15		New EU countries since 2004		Israel, Norway and Switzerland		South-eastern Europe		CIS		Total	
	No.	%	No.	%	No.	%	No.	%	No.	%	No.	%	No.	%
After 2005	16	59	9	60	7	58	1	33	2	29	1	20	20	48
1999–2004	7	26	5	33	2	17	1	33	3	43	3	60	14	33
Before 1998	3	11	0	0	3	25	0	0	1	14	1	20	5	12
2004[a]	0	0	0	0	0	0	0	0	1	14	0	0	1	2
Information not available	1	4	1	7	0	0	1	33	0	0	0	0	2	5

[a] Draft law prepared and submitted.

- Bulgaria: the Ministry of Health (or its regional departments) does not monitor the implementation of mental health legislation, only nongovernmental organizations. As reported, guardianship is often arbitrarily used for people with mental disabilities.
- Georgia: although the Law on Psychiatric Care reflects the basic rights and principles of modern psychiatric care, it is not implemented effectively due to insufficient funding from government and the absence of mechanisms for law enforcement; further, the relevant training and supervision of the mental health services personnel, police and judicial or criminal justice institutions have not taken place to promote understanding of the Law.
- The former Yugoslav Republic of Macedonia: for many years, the involuntary hospitalization procedure was covered by the Law for Non-litigation Procedure, which is obsolete, and the monitoring and inspection practices are covered by the new Law on Mental Health from 2006. More importantly, there is a total lack of implementation regarding both the involuntary hospitalization procedure and the monitoring.

Fig. 3.2. The year of the last version of the approved mental health legislation in countries

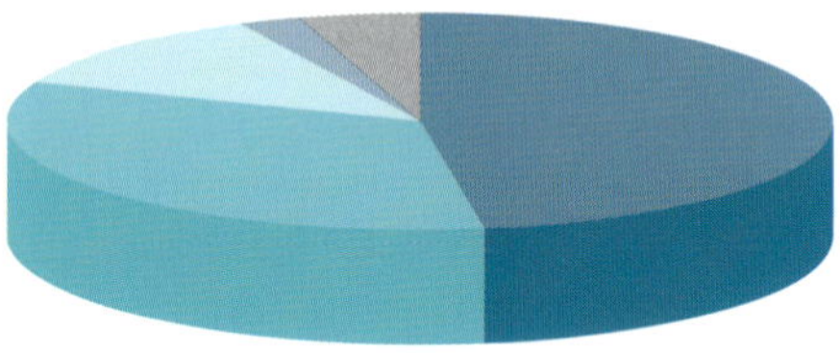

After 2005:
Austria, Belgium, Bulgaria, Czech Republic, Denmark, Estonia, Finland, France, Georgia, Germany, Ireland, Italy, Latvia, Lithuania, Montenegro, Norway, Poland, Slovakia, Spain (Castilla y León), the former Yugoslav Republic of Macedonia, United Kingdom (England and Wales)

1999–2004:
Azerbaijan, Bosnia and Herzegovina (Federation of Bosnia and Herzegovina and Republika Srpska), Croatia, Cyprus, Greece, Israel, Netherlands, Portugal, Romania, Russian Federation, Spain, Spain (Catalonia, Extremadura and Murcia), Sweden, Turkey, United Kingdom (Scotland), Uzbekistan

Before 1998:
Albania, Hungary, Malta, Moldova, Slovenia, Spain (Galicia)

Draft law prepared and submitted to the Ministry of Health in 2004:
Serbia

Information not available:
Luxembourg, Switzerland

Discussion

Activity in policy and legislation has flourished in recent years. Since 2005, 57% of countries have adopted new mental health policies and 48% have introduced new legislation. Only four countries do not yet have a strategy. Only five of the countries still have legislation that is more than 10 years old.

Most countries have opted for a separate mental health strategy, but many have included mental health within their overall health policy documents. The same applies to legislation. Determining the merits of the respective approaches would require detailed content analysis, which is well beyond the scope of this report. The advantages of an integrated strategy are avoiding the fragmentation and isolation of mental health; the advantages of a separate document are greater flexibility and visibility.

Most countries indicate that policy and legislation contain most of the subjects that should be covered. A concern is that guardianship, capacity and family rights are lacking in the legislation in some countries. The lack of attention to the rights of carers is also of concern. A good case can be made that guardianship and capacity are issues beyond the confines of mental health legislation, particularly essential for protecting the human rights of people with intellectual disability, and many countries have such legislation. The question is therefore not whether mental health legislation includes such protection but whether such general legislation covers people with mental health problems. This question was beyond the scope of this report.

Strategies and legislation tend to be given great importance, and they are an important foundation for the development of mental health systems. However, some perspective is necessary. Policies can be compared to cookbooks. Without a good recipe, bread may turn out rather awkward, although well-trained cooks will produce some nice bread anyway. Sweden may be an example, not having a recent strategy but decent services. However, a good recipe on its own produces no food but can result in lots of discussions about food. Ingredients, ovens, heat and cooks are necessary.

Committed experts are spending considerable time drafting policies in many parts of the Region, often making considerable impact. However, in some countries, desks in ministries are collapsing under the weight of policies that have never been implemented. Sometimes the reason is that the policies that have been drafted are politically unacceptable and are therefore not adopted. However, many ambitious strategies are accepted by ministers, governments and even parliaments but still not implemented. In the countries that lack the political will, planners and psychiatrists do not comply with legislation, which is subsequently ignored. Even the many countries with genuine commitment to the implementation of modern community-based mental health services face challenges in implementation. The obstacles can be the absence of skilled leaders, a competent workforce, infrastructure, partnerships and/or funding. The Mental Health Declaration for Europe specifies the essential components of mental health policies and programmes, and the other chapters in this report scrutinize the state of development in European countries.

Table 3.4. Content and components included in mental health legislation in countries

Country	Access to mental health care	Access to care in community settings	Legal rights of mental health service users	Legal rights of family members of mental health service users and other carers	Competency or capacity issues for people with mental illness	Guardianship issues for people with mental illness	Mechanisms to oversee involuntary admission	Voluntary and involuntary treatment, procedures and safeguards	Accreditation of professionals	Accreditation of facilities	Law enforcement and other judicial system issues for people with mental illness	Mechanisms to monitor involuntary treatment practices	Mechanisms to implement the provisions of mental health legislation
Albania	Yes	Yes	Yes	No	Yes	Yes	Yes	Yes	No	No	Yes	Yes	Yes
Austria	No	No	Yes	Yes	Yes	Yes	Yes	Yes	Yes	Yes	Yes	Yes	No
Azerbaijan	Yes	Yes	Yes	No	Yes	Yes	Yes	Yes	Yes	Yes	Yes	No	No
Belgium	Yes	Yes	Yes	Yes	Yes	Yes	Yes	Yes	Yes	Yes	Yes	Yes	Yes
Bosnia and Herzegovina	Information not available	Information not available	Information not available	Information not available	Information not available	Information not available	Information not available	Information not available	Information not available	Information not available	Information not available	Information not available	Information not available
Federation of Bosnia and Herzegovina	Yes	Yes	Yes	Yes	Yes	Yes	Yes	Yes	Yes	Yes	Yes	Yes	Yes
Republika Srpska	Yes	Yes	Yes	Yes	Yes	Yes	Yes	Yes	Yes	Yes	Yes	Yes	Yes
Bulgaria	Yes	Yes	Yes	No	Yes	No	Yes	Yes	No	Yes	No	No	No
Croatia	Yes	Yes	Yes	Yes	Yes	Yes	Yes	Yes	Yes	Yes	Yes	Yes	Yes
Cyprus	No	No	Yes	Yes	Yes	Yes	Yes	Yes	No	No	Yes	Yes	Yes
Czech Republic	No	No	Yes	Yes	Yes	No	Yes	Yes	Yes	Yes	Yes	Yes	No
Denmark	Yes	Yes	Yes	Yes	Yes	Yes	Yes	Yes	Yes	Yes	Yes	Yes	Yes
Estonia	No	No	Yes	No	No	No	Yes	Yes	No	No	Yes	No	No
Finland	Yes	Yes	Yes	No	No	No	Yes	Yes	No	No	No	Yes	Yes
France	Yes	Yes	Yes	Yes	Yes	Yes	Yes	Yes	Yes	Yes	Yes	Yes	Yes
Georgia	Yes	No	Yes	No	Yes	No	Yes	Yes	No	No	No	Yes	No
Germany	Yes	Yes	Yes	Yes	Yes	Yes	Yes	Yes	Yes	Yes	Yes	Yes	Yes
Greece	Yes	Yes	Yes	No	No	No	No	Yes	No	No	No	No	No
Hungary	Yes	Yes	Yes	Yes	Yes	Yes	Yes	Yes	Yes	Yes	Yes	Yes	Yes
Ireland	No	No	Yes	No	No	No	Yes	Yes	No	Yes	Yes	Yes	Yes
Israel	Yes	Yes	Yes	No	Yes	Yes	Yes	Yes	Yes	Yes	Yes	Yes	Yes
Italy	Yes	Yes	Yes	No	Yes	Yes	Yes	Yes	Yes	Yes	Yes	Yes	Yes
Latvia	Yes	Yes	Yes	Yes	Yes	Yes	Yes	Yes	Yes	Yes	Yes	Yes	Yes
Lithuania	Yes	Yes	Yes	Yes	Yes	No	Yes	Yes	No	No	Yes	Yes	No
Luxembourg	Yes	Yes	Yes	Yes	Yes	Yes	Yes	Yes	Yes	Yes	Yes	Yes	No
Malta	Yes	Yes	Yes	Yes	Yes	Yes	Yes	Yes	No	Yes	Yes	Yes	Yes
Moldova	Yes	No	Yes	No	No	Yes	Yes	Yes	No	No	Yes	Yes	No
Montenegro	Yes	Yes	Yes	Yes	Yes	No	Yes	Yes	Yes	Yes	Yes	Yes	Yes
Netherlands	No	No	Yes	Yes	Yes	Yes	Yes	Yes	Yes	Yes	Yes	Yes	Yes

Yes ■ No ■ Information not available

Table 3.4. continued

Country	Access to mental health care	Access to care in community settings	Legal rights of mental health service users	Legal rights of family members of mental health service users and other carers	Competency or capacity issues for people with mental illness	Guardianship issues for people with mental illness	Mechanisms to oversee involuntary admission	Voluntary and involuntary treatment, procedures and safeguards	Accreditation of professionals	Accreditation of facilities	Law enforcement and other judicial system issues for people with mental illness	Mechanisms to monitor involuntary treatment practices	Mechanisms to implement the provisions of mental health legislation
Norway	Yes	Yes	Yes	Yes	Yes	Yes	Yes	Yes	Yes	Yes	Yes	Yes	Yes
Poland	Yes	Yes	Yes	Yes	Yes	Yes	Yes	Yes	Yes	Yes	Yes	Yes	Yes
Portugal	Yes	Yes	Yes	Yes	Yes	No	Yes	Yes	Yes	No	Yes	Yes	No
Romania	Yes	Yes	Yes	No	Yes	Yes	Yes	Yes	Yes	No	Yes	Yes	Yes
Russian Federation	Yes	Yes	Yes	Yes	Yes	Yes	Yes	Yes	Yes	Yes	Yes	Yes	Yes
Serbia	No	No	No	No	No	No	No	No	No	No	No	No	No
Slovakia	Yes	Yes	Yes	Yes	Yes	Yes	Yes	Yes	Information not available	Information not available	No	No	No
Slovenia	No	No	No	No	Yes	Yes	No	Yes	Yes	Yes	Yes	Yes	No
Spain	No	No	No	No	Yes	Yes	Yes	Yes	Yes	No	No	No	No
Castilla y León	Yes	Yes	Yes	Yes	Yes	Yes	Yes	Yes	Yes	No	No	Yes	Yes
Catalonia	Yes	Yes	Yes	No	Yes	Yes	Yes	Yes	Yes	Yes	Information not available	Yes	Yes
Extremadura	Yes	Yes	Yes	No	Yes	Yes	Yes	Yes	Yes	Yes	Information not available	Yes	Information not available
Galicia	Yes	Yes	No	No	No	No	No	No	No	Yes	No	No	No
Murcia	Yes	Yes	Yes	No	Yes	Yes	Yes	Yes	Yes	Yes	Information not available	Yes	No
Sweden	Information not available	Information not available	Information not available	Information not available	Information not available	Information not available	Information not available	Information not available	Information not available	Information not available	Information not available	Information not available	Information not available
Switzerland	Yes	Yes	Yes	No	Yes	Yes	Information not available	Yes	Yes	Yes	Information not available	No	No
The former Yugoslav Republic of Macedonia	Yes	Yes	Yes	Yes	No	No	No	Yes	No	No	No	Yes	Yes
Turkey	Yes	Yes	Yes	Yes	Yes	Yes	Yes	Yes	No	No	Yes	Yes	Yes
United Kingdom													
England and Wales	Yes	Yes	Yes	Yes	Yes	Yes	Yes	Yes	Yes	Yes	Yes	Yes	Yes
Scotland	Yes	Yes	Yes	Yes	Yes	Yes	Yes	Yes	Yes	No	Yes	Yes	Yes
Uzbekistan	Yes	Yes	Yes	Yes	Yes	Yes	Yes	Yes	Yes	Yes	Yes	Yes	Yes

Yes ■ No ■ Information not available

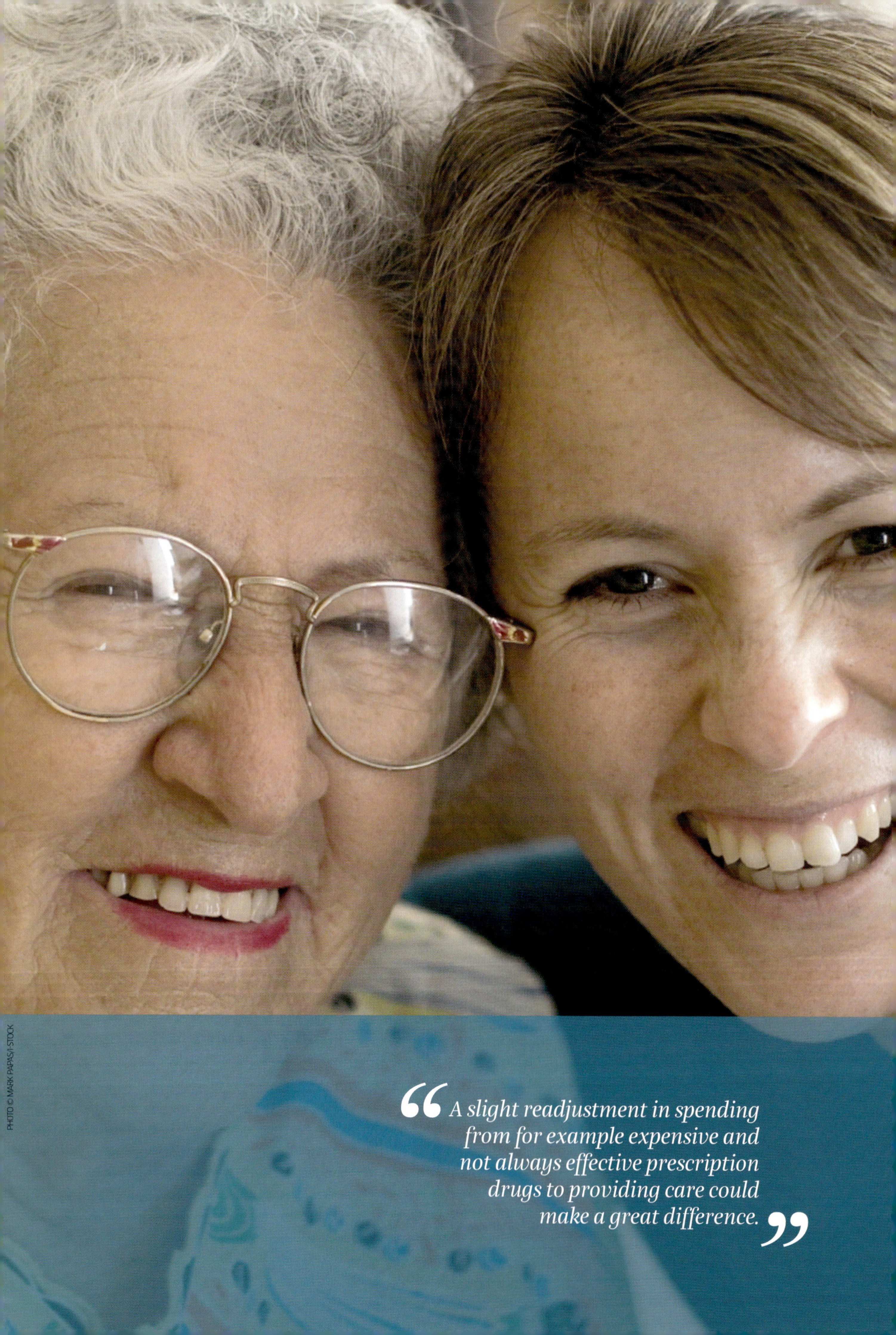

PHOTO © MARK PAPAS/ISTOCK

“A slight readjustment in spending from for example expensive and not always effective prescription drugs to providing care could make a great difference.”

4. Promoting mental health and preventing mental disorders

The Mental Health Declaration for Europe and Mental Health Action Plan for Europe identify promoting mental health, reducing stigma, discrimination and social exclusion and preventing mental health problems as priorities for the next decade. A lack of awareness of the importance of mental well-being for the individual and for the society as a whole increases the risk of mental ill health for vulnerable population groups. A lack of knowledge about mental disorders, their symptoms and responsiveness to treatment often lead to prejudices towards people with mental illness and subsequently to stigmatization, social exclusion and discrimination.

Promoting mental health, reducing stigmatization and preventing mental disorders have been shown to be effective in reducing the burden of mental disorders. Member States assumed responsibilities to deliver on this priority at national level and committed themselves:

- to promote mental health in education and employment, communities and other relevant settings;
- to eliminate stigma and discrimination and enhance inclusion by increasing public awareness;
- to prevent risk factors in relevant settings and to address the prevention of suicide and depression; and
- to consider the potential impact of all public policies on mental health.

> **Definitions**
>
> Mental health promotion aims to protect, support and sustain emotional and social well-being and create individual, social and environmental conditions that enable optimal psychological and psychophysiological development and improve the coping capacity of individuals. Mental health promotion refers to positive mental health rather than mental ill health.
>
> A stigma is a distinguishing mark establishing a demarcation between the stigmatized person and others attributing negative characteristics to this person. The stigma attached to mental illness often leads to social exclusion and discrimination and creates an additional burden for the affected individual.
>
> Mental disorder prevention focuses on reducing risk factors and enhancing protective factors associated with mental ill health with the aim of reducing the risk, incidence, prevalence and recurrence of mental disorders.

Promoting mental health and tackling stigma and discrimination

Raising public awareness

According to the responses, almost all countries have implemented programmes and/or activities to raise public awareness about mental health and mental disorders during the past five years (Table 4.1).

Programmes and activities range widely, including participation in huge networks such as the European Alliance against Depression, national programmes such as See Me in the United Kingdom (Scotland), local television and radio broadcasts and single awareness-raising events.

Of the 36 countries indicating that programmes have been implemented, only 7 said that the activities have been evaluated and the results of evaluation are available. The evaluations show an overall positive effect in terms of raising awareness and sensitivity for mental health–related topics.

Five countries said that no programmes and/or activities have been implemented during the past five years.

In most of the countries, nongovernmental organizations or government agencies have promoted programmes and activities (Table 4.2). International agencies have been particularly active in countries in south-eastern Europe and CIS countries.

Table 4.1. Implementation of programmes and/or activities to raise public awareness about mental health and mental disorders during the past five years in groups of countries

	EU		EU15		New EU countries since 2004		Israel, Norway and Switzerland		South-eastern Europe		CIS		Total	
Implementation	No.	%	No.	%	No.	%	No.	%	No.	%	No.	%	No.	%
Yes	24	89	13	87	11	92	3	100	6	86	3	60	36	86
No	2	7	1	7	1	8	0	0	1	14	2	40	5	12
Information not available	1	4	1	7	0	0	0	0	0	0	0	0	1	2

Table 4.2. Extent to which agencies, institutions or services have promoted public education and awareness campaigns on mental health and mental disorders during the past five years in groups of countries

	EU		EU15		New EU countries since 2004		Israel, Norway and Switzerland		South-eastern Europe		CIS		Total	
Promoters of campaigns	No.	%	No.	%	No.	%	No.	%	No.	%	No.	%	No.	%
Government agencies[a]														
Yes	22	81	13	87	9	75	3	100	6	86	3	60	34	81
No	5	19	2	13	3	25	0	0	1	14	2	40	8	19
Nongovernmental organizations														
Yes	24	89	13	87	11	92	3	100	6	86	4	80	37	88
No	2	7	1	7	1	8	0	0	0	0	1	20	3	7
No information available	1	4	1	7	0	0	0	0	1	14	0	0	2	5
Professional associations														
Yes	15	56	9	60	6	50	3	100	5	71	4	80	27	64
No	6	22	1	7	5	42	0	0	1	14	1	20	8	19
No information available	6	22	5	33	1	8	0	0	1	14	0	0	7	17
Private trusts and foundations														
Yes	13	48	7	47	6	50	1	33	3	43	1	20	18	43
No	6	22	2	13	4	33	1	33	2	29	3	60	12	29
No information available	8	30	6	40	2	17	1	33	2	29	1	20	12	29
International agencies														
Yes	11	41	7	47	4	33	0	0	6	86	4	80	21	50
No	8	30	3	20	5	42	0	0	0	0	1	20	9	21
No information available	8	30	5	33	3	25	3	100	1	14	0	0	12	29

[a] Such as the ministry of health or department of mental health services.

Tackling stigma and discrimination

Programmes and/or activities to tackle stigma and discrimination against people with mental health problems have been implemented in 83% of the countries (Fig. 4.1). Almost all EU countries, 71% of the countries in south-eastern Europe and 40% of the CIS countries participating in the survey indicated programmes and/or activities (Table 4.3).

Similar to mental health promotion, there is a wide range of anti-stigma activities. There are campaigns carried out by organizations of carers such as Zero Stigma in several European countries, national campaigns such as Shift in the United Kingdom (England and Wales) as well as partnerships within Open the Doors, the global anti-stigma programme of the World Psychiatric Association in Germany, Greece, Italy, Poland and Slovakia. There are also local initiatives such as anti-stigma seminars for health professionals about the human rights situation in mental health services and the needs of service users in Latvia.

Few countries reported about evaluation of activities. Where evaluation has taken place, an overall reduction of stigma as a result from the activities has been reported. Zero Stigma in Austria placed 30 000 free cards at public places in Vienna, carried out by the Austrian carer organization HPE (Hilfe für Angehörige und Freunde psychisch Erkrankter) with the support of the European Federation of Associations of Families of People with Mental Illness. This activity led to an increased number of visits at the web site, numerous e-mail enquiries and increased distribution of information booklets. The Bavarian Anti-stigma Action (BASTA) in Germany evaluated workshops with police officers. Attitudes towards people with mental disorders have improved and the social distance towards them has declined. Open the Doors Düsseldorf in Germany has reduced social distance in the general public by implementing the global anti-stigma programme of the World Psychiatric Association at various levels and in different target groups over years. See Me in the United Kingdom (Scotland) has been thoroughly evaluated (see http://www.seemescotland.org.uk for its methods and results).

Nongovernmental organizations and government agencies have initiated most of the anti-stigma activities (Table 4.4).

Table 4.3. Implementation of programmes and/or activities to tackle stigma and discrimination against people with mental disorders during the past five years in groups of countries

	EU		EU15		New EU countries since 2004		Israel, Norway and Switzerland		South-eastern Europe		CIS		Total	
Implementation	No.	%	No.	%	No.	%	No.	%	No.	%	No.	%	No.	%
Yes	25	93	13	87	12	100	3	100	5	71	2	40	35	83
No	0	0	0	0	0	0	0	0	2	29	3	60	5	12
Information not available	2	7	2	13	0	0	0	0	0	0	0	0	2	5

Table 4.4. Extent to which agencies, institutions or services have run activities to tackle stigma and discrimination against people with mental disorders during the past five years in groups of countries

Implementers of activities	EU		EU15		New EU countries since 2004		Israel, Norway and Switzerland		South-eastern Europe		CIS		Total	
	No.	%	No.	%	No.	%	No.	%	No.	%	No.	%	No.	%
Government agencies[a]														
Yes	16	59	8	53	8	67	3	100	5	71	3	60	27	64
No	6	22	4	27	2	17	0	0	2	29	2	40	10	24
No information available	5	19	3	20	2	17	0	0	0	0	0	0	5	12
Nongovernmental organizations														
Yes	24	89	12	80	12	100	3	100	4	57	3	60	34	81
No	1	4	1	7	0	0	0	0	2	29	2	40	5	12
No information available	2	7	2	13	0	0	0	0	1	14	0	0	3	7
Professional associations														
Yes	9	33	6	40	3	25	2	67	2	29	2	40	15	36
No	10	37	4	27	6	50	0	0	3	43	3	60	16	38
No information available	8	30	5	33	3	25	1	33	2	29	0	0	11	26
Private trusts and foundations														
Yes	12	44	9	60	3	25	2	67	2	29	1	20	17	40
No	5	19	1	7	4	33	0	0	3	43	3	60	11	26
No information available	10	37	5	33	5	42	1	33	2	29	1	20	14	33
International agencies														
Yes	6	22	4	27	2	17	0	0	3	43	4	80	13	31
No	8	30	3	20	5	42	0	0	2	29	1	20	11	26
No information available	13	48	8	53	5	42	3	100	2	29	0	0	18	43

[a] Such as the ministry of health or department of mental health services.

Fig. 4.1. Programmes and/or activities to tackle stigma and discrimination in countries

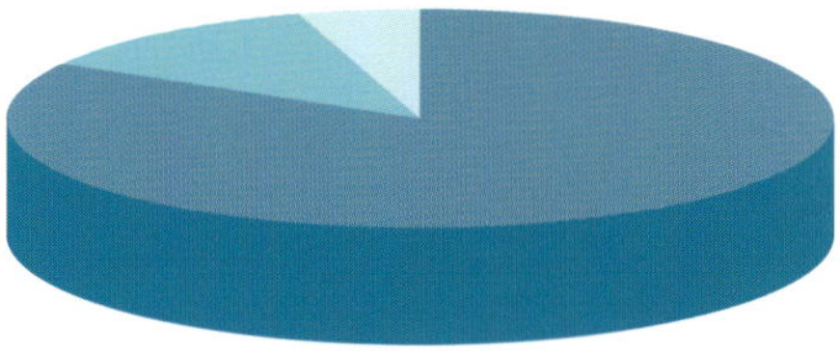

Yes:
Albania, Austria, Belgium, Bosnia and Herzegovina (Federation of Bosnia and Herzegovina and Republika Srpska), Bulgaria, Croatia, Cyprus, Czech Republic, Denmark, Estonia, Finland, France, Georgia, Germany, Greece, Hungary, Israel, Italy, Latvia, Lithuania, Luxembourg, Malta, Netherlands, Norway, Poland, Romania, Russian Federation, Serbia, Slovakia, Slovenia, Spain (Castilla y León, Catalonia, Extremadura and Galicia), Sweden, Switzerland, the former Yugoslav Republic of Macedonia, United Kingdom (England and Wales and Scotland)

No:
Azerbaijan, Montenegro, Moldova, Spain (Murcia), Turkey, Uzbekistan

Information not available:
Ireland, Portugal

Mental health promotion programmes and activities

Almost forty per cent of the countries indicate that programmes to improve parenting have been implemented during the past five years in all or in the majority of community settings. Most of the activities mentioned to improve parenting have been implemented over a longer period, are still ongoing and, in some cases, are integrated in national policy and government action plans (Table 4.5).

In Austria, several nongovernmental organizations have carried out the parenting skills training programme Elternbildung with support from the Federal Ministry of Health, Family and Youth. It has been implemented in all nine provinces to promote nonviolent education and to prevent problems in familial relationships.

Centres for social services for children and families have been established in 10 large cities in Bulgaria since 2006 in the framework of the EU-funded project Reform for Improving the Well-being of Children. The centres provide consultations for families at risk and future foster parents and adoptive parents.

In Germany, a national Prevention Prize (€50 000) under the motto "Enhancing the Competency of Parents during Pregnancy and Early Childhood" was awarded in 2006.

Programmes to promote the mental health of children and adolescents are available in more than half the schools in more than 40% of the countries. The activities range from workshops on conflict resolution and social and emotional learning to overarching programmes that address several topics specific to target groups. Six countries responded that they have no promotion activities in schools (Table 4.6).

Table 4.5. Implementation of programmes and/or activities to improve parenting during the past five years in groups of countries

Programmes and/or activities implemented in community or home-based settings	EU		EU15		New EU countries since 2004		Israel, Norway and Switzerland		South-eastern Europe		CIS		Total	
	No.	%	No.	%	No.	%	No.	%	No.	%	No.	%	No.	%
Yes														
All or most (81–100%)	8	30	5	33	3	25	1	33	1	14	1	20	11	26
Majority (51–80%)	3	11	1	7	2	17	1	33	1	14	0	0	5	12
Some (21–50%)	3	11	3	20	0	0	1	33	1	14	2	40	7	17
A few (1–20%)	6	22	2	13	4	33	0	0	1	14	1	20	8	19
No (0%)	0	0	0	0	0	0	0	0	3	43	1	20	4	10
Information not available	7	26	4	27	3	25	0	0	0	0	0	0	7	17

Table 4.6. Implementation of programmes and/or activities in schools to promote the mental health of children and adolescents during the past five years in groups of countries

Programmes and/or activities implemented in schools	EU		EU15		New EU countries since 2004		Israel, Norway and Switzerland		South-eastern Europe		CIS		Total	
	No.	%	No.	%	No.	%	No.	%	No.	%	No.	%	No.	%
Yes														
All or most (81–100%)	2	7	0	0	2	17	0	0	1	14	1	20	4	10
Majority (51–80%)	8	30	5	33	3	25	2	67	2	29	1	20	13	31
Some (21–50%)	2	7	1	7	1	8	1	33	2	29	0	0	5	12
A few (1–20%)	11	41	6	40	5	42	0	0	1	14	1	20	13	31
No (0%)	3	11	2	13	1	8	0	0	1	14	2	40	6	14
Information not available	1	4	1	7	0	0	0	0	0	0	0	0	1	2

Austria implemented Eigenständig werden (Promoting Independence), a programme that combines personality development, health promotion, promoting life skills and preventing addiction and violence in primary schools among children 6–10 years old in about 600 schools by 2006. The Austrian Health Promotion Foundation co-funded this.

In contrast to the findings about the relatively high availability of school programmes, few countries indicate programmes and/or activities to promote mental health at the workplace. Only Belgium, the Netherlands, Norway and Slovenia report that activities are available in all or most workplaces. Twenty-six of the 42 countries report no promotion activities or only in 1–20% of workplaces. The available activities focus on managing stress and preventing burnout and bullying. Almost no activities have been evaluated according to the responses from countries (Table 4.7).

The results for promoting the mental health of older people were similar to those in the workplace. Only 4 of 42 countries have activities reaching all or almost all older people: Denmark, Luxembourg, Spain (Catalonia) and the United Kingdom (Scotland). More than half the countries have no or few programmes available. The implemented activities focus on physical activity, self-help and memory training (Table 4.8).

In all three areas, raising public awareness, tackling stigma and discrimination and mental health promotion, countries indicated that conducting public campaigns, working with the mass media, holding high-level expert meetings and involving governments as the main activities initiated and developed since 2005.

Table 4.7. Implementation of programmes and/or activities to promote mental health at the workplace during the past five years in groups of countries

Programmes and/or activities implemented in the workplace	EU		EU15		New EU countries since 2004		Israel, Norway and Switzerland		South-eastern Europe		CIS		Total	
	No.	%	No.	%	No.	%	No.	%	No.	%	No.	%	No.	%
Yes														
All or most (81–100%)	1	4	1	7	0	0	1	33	0	0	0	0	2	5
Majority (51–80%)	2	7	1	7	1	8	0	0	0	0	0	0	2	5
Some (21–50%)	5	19	4	27	1	8	0	0	2	29	0	0	1	17
A few (1–20%)	12	44	6	40	6	50	1	33	1	14	3	60	17	40
No (0%)	4	15	2	13	2	17	0	0	3	43	2	40	9	21
Information not available	3	11	1	7	2	17	1	33	1	14	0	0	5	12

Table 4.8. Implementation of programmes and/or activities to promote the mental health of older people during the past five years in groups of countries

Programmes and/or activities reaching older people	EU		EU15		New EU countries since 2004		Israel, Norway and Switzerland		South-eastern Europe		CIS		Total	
	No.	%	No.	%	No.	%	No.	%	No.	%	No.	%	No.	%
Yes														
All or almost all (81–100%)	4	15	4	27	0	0	0	0	0	0	0	0	4	10
Some (21–50%)	5	19	4	27	1	8	0	0	1	14	1	20	7	17
A few (1–20%)	11	41	5	33	6	50	2	67	3	43	1	20	17	40
None (0%)	3	11	0	0	3	25	0	0	2	29	2	40	7	17
Information not available	4	15	2	13	2	17	1	33	1	14	1	20	7	17

Preventing mental disorders

Policies and programmes implemented during the past five years

Eleven of the 42 countries have introduced policies to prevent suicide during the past five years by reducing access to lethal means. Programmes have been implemented in 11 countries (Table 4.9).

Policies to improve the recognition and treatment of population groups at risk in primary health care have been introduced in 15 countries and programmes in 19. Similar results have been found for policies and programmes to prevent suicide by recognizing and treating population groups at risk in specialized care: policies have been implemented in 13 countries and programmes in 18 (Tables 4.10 and 4.11).

Fourteen countries have policies to prevent depression directed towards the whole population and 17 have programmes (Table 4.12).

More of the EU countries have implemented depression prevention programmes than policies.

Programmes and activities to prevent depression show greater diversity of interventions and target groups than health promotion or anti-stigma programmes do. Austria, Germany and Spain (Catalonia) are partners in the European Alliance against Depression. Bosnia and Herzegovina (Federation of Bosnia and Herzegovina), Czech Republic and Israel reported specific mass-media campaigns and other close collaboration with the mass media. Latvia implemented a

Table 4.9. Implementation of policies or programmes to prevent suicide by reducing access to lethal means during the past five years in groups of countries

Policies and programmes implemented	EU		EU15		New EU countries since 2004		Israel, Norway and Switzerland		South-eastern Europe		CIS		Total	
	No.	%	No.	%	No.	%	No.	%	No.	%	No.	%	No.	%
Policies														
Yes	5	19	3	20	2	17	2	67	3	43	1	20	11	26
No	19	70	11	73	8	67	1	33	4	57	4	80	28	67
Information not available	3	11	1	7	2	17	0	0	0	0	0	0	3	7
Programmes														
Yes	8	30	7	47	1	8	2	67	1	14	0	0	11	26
No	16	59	7	47	9	75	1	33	6	86	4	80	27	64
Information not available	3	11	1	7	2	17	0	0	0	0	1	20	4	10

Table 4.10. Implementation of policies and programmes to prevent suicide by recognition and treatment of population groups at risk in primary health care during the past five years in groups of countries

Policies and programmes implemented	EU		EU15		New EU countries since 2004		Israel, Norway and Switzerland		South-eastern Europe		CIS		Total	
	No.	%	No.	%	No.	%	No.	%	No.	%	No.	%	No.	%
Policies														
Yes	8	30	7	47	1	8	3	100	3	43	1	20	15	36
No	18	67	8	53	10	83	0	0	4	57	4	80	26	62
Information not available	1	4	0	0	1	8	0	0	0	0	0	0	1	2
Programmes														
Yes	12	44	8	53	4	33	1	33	4	57	2	40	19	45
No	14	52	7	47	7	58	1	33	3	43	3	60	21	50
Information not available	1	4	0	0	1	8	1	33	0	0	0	0	2	5

crisis phone line. In Belgium and especially in the Flemish region, a public campaign for the primary prevention of depression: Fit in je hoofd, goed in je vel (Fit in your head, good in your skin) has been run, offering a web site with exercises for mental fitness for preventing depression.

In Germany, a Competency Network for Depression and Suicidality has been established, a national network aimed at optimizing research and care related to depressive disorders funded by the Federal Ministry for Education and Research.

Table 4.11. Implementation of policies and programmes to prevent suicide by recognition and treatment of population groups at risk in specialized care during the past five years in groups of countries

Policies and programmes implemented	EU		EU15		New EU countries since 2004		Israel, Norway and Switzerland		South-eastern Europe		CIS		Total	
	No.	%	No.	%	No.	%	No.	%	No.	%	No.	%	No.	%
Policies														
Yes	7	26	6	40	1	8	1	33	4	57	1	20	13	31
No	19	70	9	60	10	83	1	33	3	43	4	80	27	64
Information not available	1	4	0	0	1	8	1	33	0	0	0	0	2	5
Programmes														
Yes	13	48	8	53	5	42	1	33	2	29	2	40	18	43
No	13	48	7	47	6	50	2	67	5	71	3	60	23	55
Information not available	1	4	0	0	1	8	0	0	0	0	0	0	1	2

Table 4.12. Implementation of policies and programmes to prevent depression directed towards the whole population during the past five years in groups of countries

Policies and programmes implemented	EU		EU15		New EU countries since 2004		Israel, Norway and Switzerland		South-eastern Europe		CIS		Total	
	No.	%	No.	%	No.	%	No.	%	No.	%	No.	%	No.	%
Policies														
Yes	10	37	9	60	1	8	1	33	1	14	2	40	14	33
No	14	52	4	27	10	83	2	67	6	86	3	60	25	60
Information not available	3	11	2	13	1	8	0	0	0	0	0	0	3	7
Programmes														
Yes	13	48	9	60	4	33	2	67	1	14	1	20	17	40
No	12	44	5	33	7	58	1	33	6	86	4	80	23	55
Information not available	2	7	1	7	1	8	0	0	0	0	0	0	2	5

Of the 42 countries, 7 have introduced policies and 11 countries programmes targeting the children of mentally ill parents or other children at risk. Policies addressing women at risk (such as preventing postpartum depression) have been implemented in 6 countries and programmes in 14 countries. For employees at risk, only four countries have introduced policies and eight countries programmes. Five countries have implemented policies to improve bereavement and support for widows and widowers and eight countries programmes (Tables 4.13–4.16).

Two thirds of the countries have implemented policies or programmes to prevent mental disorders among population groups that are at risk or vulnerable. Many of the activities target refugees. Denmark has specialized centres for treating traumatized refugees who have post-traumatic stress syndrome, day care centres and hostels for refugees with mental illness have been established in Greece and the former Yugoslav Republic of Macedonia reports a project to support Roma refugees from Kosovo (Table 4.17). Serbia had several programmes:

- preventing mental disorders among refugees (supported by the Office of the United Nations High Commissioner for Refugees (UNHCR) from 1993 to 2000);
- preventing mental disorders among ex-detainees (2000) supported by the Norwegian Committee for Human Rights;
- the Centre for Rehabilitation of Torture Victims, which was started by the nongovernmental organization IAN (International Aid Network) and supported by the European Commission (2000–2004);

Table 4.13. Implementation of policies and programmes to prevent depression among children of mentally ill parents (or other children at risk) during the past five years in groups of countries

Policies and programmes implemented	EU		EU15		New EU countries since 2004		Israel, Norway and Switzerland		South-eastern Europe		CIS		Total	
	No.	%	No.	%	No.	%	No.	%	No.	%	No.	%	No.	%
Policies														
Yes	5	19	5	33	0	0	1	33	1	14	0	0	7	17
No	19	70	8	53	11	92	2	67	6	86	5	100	32	76
Information not available	3	11	2	13	1	8	0	0	0	0	0	0	3	7
Programmes														
Yes	8	30	7	47	1	8	2	67	1	14	0	0	11	26
No	17	63	7	47	10	83	1	33	6	86	5	100	29	69
Information not available	2	7	1	7	1	8	0	0	0	0	0	0	2	5

Table 4.14. Implementation of policies and programmes to prevent depression among women at risk (such as preventing postpartum depression) during the past five years in groups of countries

Policies and programmes implemented	EU		EU15		New EU countries since 2004		Israel, Norway and Switzerland		South-eastern Europe		CIS		Total	
	No.	%	No.	%	No.	%	No.	%	No.	%	No.	%	No.	%
Policies														
Yes	4	15	4	27	0	0	1	33	1	14	0	0	6	14
No	20	74	9	60	11	92	2	67	6	86	5	100	33	79
Information not available	3	11	2	13	1	8	0	0	0	0	0	0	3	7
Programmes														
Yes	10	37	8	53	2	17	1	33	1	14	2	40	14	33
No	15	56	6	40	9	75	2	67	6	86	3	60	26	62
Information not available	2	7	1	7	1	8	0	0	0	0	0	0	2	5

Table 4.15. Implementation of policies and programmes to prevent depression among employees at risk during the past five years in groups of countries

Policies and programmes implemented	EU		EU15		New EU countries since 2004		Israel, Norway and Switzerland		South-eastern Europe		CIS		Total	
	No.	%	No.	%	No.	%	No.	%	No.	%	No.	%	No.	%
Policies														
Yes	3	11	3	20	0	0	0	0	1	14	0	0	4	10
No	21	78	10	67	11	92	3	100	6	86	5	100	35	83
Information not available	3	11	2	13	1	8	0	0	0	0	0	0	3	7
Programmes														
Yes	5	19	4	27	1	8	1	33	1	14	1	20	8	19
No	19	70	9	60	10	83	2	67	6	86	4	80	31	74
Information not available	3	11	2	13	1	8	0	0	0	0	0	0	3	7

Table 4.16. Implementation of policies and programmes to prevent depression related to bereavement and to support widows and widowers during the past five years in groups of countries

Policies and programmes implemented	EU		EU15		New EU countries since 2004		Israel, Norway and Switzerland		South-eastern Europe		CIS		Total	
	No.	%	No.	%	No.	%	No.	%	No.	%	No.	%	No.	%
Policies														
Yes	3	11	3	20	0	0	1	33	1	14	0	0	5	12
No	21	78	10	67	11	92	2	67	6	86	5	100	34	81
Information not available	3	11	2	13	1	8	0	0	0	0	0	0	3	7
Programmes														
Yes	5	19	5	33	0	0	1	33	1	14	1	20	8	19
No	19	70	8	53	11	92	2	67	6	86	4	80	31	74
Information not available	3	11	2	13	1	8	0	0	0	0	0	0	3	7

- programmes for preventing mental disorders among older people, children and adolescents (supported by the United Nations Children's Fund (UNICEF));
- preventing child abuse (supported by Intercare the Netherlands); and
- preventing mental disorders among internally displaced people.

Mental health specialists are available in schools in more than half the countries, and teachers are trained in identifying mental health problems in one third of the countries. The mental health specialists are mainly school psychologists and social workers. In several countries, schools can refer children with learning problems to educational counsellors (Table 4.18).

In Ireland, all primary and post-primary schools have access to psychological assessments either directly through the National Education Psychological Service or through the Scheme for Commissioning Psychological Assessments. These agents provide a range of services to support the personal, social and educational development of children in primary and secondary schools by applying psychological theory and practice in education with particular regard for those with special education needs.

Main activities initiated and developed since 2005

The main activities initiated and developed for preventing suicide and depression since 2005 have been implementing public campaigns, working with the mass media, training health professionals, especially general practitioners (GPs), and collaborating with governments. Three countries (Belgium, Germany and the United Kingdom (England and Wales)) have integrated activities to prevent mental disorders into government action plans since 2005.

Table 4.17. Development of policies and programmes to prevent mental disorders specifically in at-risk or vulnerable population groups during the past five years in groups of countries

Policies and programmes developed	EU		EU15		New EU countries since 2004		Israel, Norway and Switzerland		South-eastern Europe		CIS		Total	
	No.	%	No.	%	No.	%	No.	%	No.	%	No.	%	No.	%
Yes	19	70	13	87	6	50	2	67	4	57	3	60	28	67
No	5	19	0	0	5	42	1	33	3	43	2	40	11	26
Information not available	3	11	2	13	1	8	0	0	0	0	0	0	3	7

Table 4.18. Procedures in place in the school setting to identify and refer children at risk for mental disorders to mental health support in groups of countries

Availability of staff in schools	EU		EU15		New EU countries since 2004		Israel, Norway and Switzerland		South-eastern Europe		CIS		Total	
	No.	%	No.	%	No.	%	No.	%	No.	%	No.	%	No.	%
Mental health specialists														
Yes	14	52	8	53	6	50	2	67	5	71	1	20	22	52
No	10	37	5	33	5	42	0	0	0	0	4	80	14	33
Information not available	3	11	2	13	1	8	1	33	2	29	0	0	6	14
Teachers trained in identification and referral														
Yes	9	33	6	40	3	25	0	0	3	43	1	20	13	31
No	9	33	4	27	5	42	1	33	4	57	4	80	18	43
Information not available	9	33	5	33	4	33	2	67	0	0	0	0	11	26

Centrality of mental health

Health impact assessment specifically including mental health is carried out in 16 of the 42 countries (Table 4.19, Fig. 4.2).

In the Czech Republic, the Institute of Health Information and Statistics has carried out a health interview survey every three years since 1993. The Danish Quality Assessment Programme is an accreditation system mandatory for both somatic and mental health hospitals. National quality assessments of the perceptions of people who have received mental health care are carried out every year. The Programme measures the quality of care provided by the hospitals to groups of people with specific disorders, such as schizophrenia.

In eight countries, policies and safety regulations that include preventing work-related stress have been developed in partnership between the employment and health sectors (Table 4.20, Fig. 4.3).

In Germany, policy-makers have anchored a series of approaches in a number of laws cutting across all departments to support prevention at the workplace. In the United Kingdom (England and Wales), national health and safety legislation includes responsibilities for protecting both physical and mental health. Regional employment teams are being developed as one action identified within Reaching Out: an Action Plan on Social Exclusion, which sets out the Government's commitment to tackle social exclusion for people with mental health problems. Lithuania reports professional risk assessment regulations, which regulate assessment of the psychosocial working environment at the workplace and prevent work-related stress.

In almost half the countries, mental health has been integrated into the school curricula through partnership work between the

Fig. 4.2. Mental health specifically included in the health impact assessment of public policies in countries

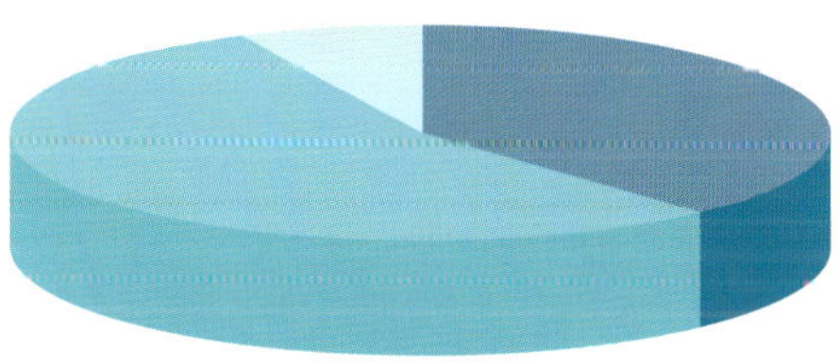

Yes:
Croatia, Czech Republic, Denmark, France, Germany, Hungary, Israel, Italy, Luxembourg, Netherlands, Norway, Poland, Russian Federation, Serbia, Spain (Castilla y León and Catalonia), Sweden, United Kingdom (England and Wales)

No:
Albania, Austria, Azerbaijan, Belgium, Bulgaria, Cyprus, Estonia, Finland, Georgia, Greece, Ireland, Latvia, Lithuania, Malta, Portugal, Moldova, Romania, Slovakia, Slovenia, Spain (Galicia), Switzerland, the former Yugoslav Republic of Macedonia, Turkey, United Kingdom (Scotland), Uzbekistan

Information not available:
Bosnia and Herzegovina (Federation of Bosnia and Herzegovina and Republika Srpska), Montenegro, Spain (Extremadura and Murcia)

Table 4.19. Specific inclusion of mental health in the health impact assessment of public policies in groups of countries

Specific inclusion	EU		EU15		New EU countries since 2004		Israel, Norway and Switzerland		South-eastern Europe		CIS		Total	
	No.	%	No.	%	No.	%	No.	%	No.	%	No.	%	No.	%
Yes	11	41	8	53	3	25	2	67	2	29	1	20	16	38
No	15	56	6	40	9	75	1	33	3	43	4	80	23	55
Information not available	1	4	1	7	0	0	0	0	2	29	0	0	3	7

Table 4.20. Development of occupational health policies and safety regulations that include preventing work-related stress in partnership by the employment and health sectors in groups of countries

Policies and safety regulations by the employment and health sectors	EU		EU15		New EU countries since 2004		Israel, Norway and Switzerland		South-eastern Europe		CIS		Total	
	No.	%	No.	%	No.	%	No.	%	No.	%	No.	%	No.	%
Yes, developed in partnership	6	22	4	27	2	17	1	33	1	14	0	0	8	19
Yes, but not developed in partnership	10	37	6	40	4	33	2	67	0	0	0	0	12	29
No such policies	8	30	4	27	4	33	0	0	4	57	4	80	16	38
Information not available	3	11	1	7	2	17	0	0	2	29	1	20	6	14

Fig. 4.3. Occupational health policies and safety regulations that include preventing work-related stress have been developed in partnership with the employment and health sectors in countries

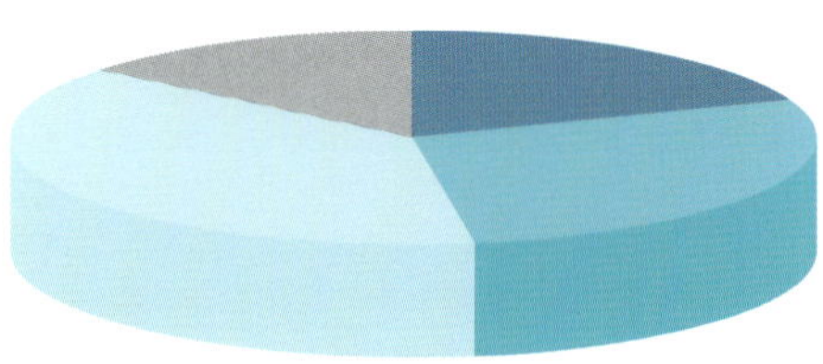

Yes, there are policies and regulations developed in partnership between the two sectors :
Austria, Croatia, Czech Republic, Finland, Germany, Norway, Romania, United Kingdom (England and Wales)

Yes, there are policies and regulations but not developed in partnership between the two sectors:
Belgium, Denmark, Estonia, France, Hungary, Israel, Italy, Latvia, Lithuania, Luxembourg, Netherlands, Switzerland

No, there are no such policies:
Albania, Azerbaijan, Cyprus, Georgia, Greece, Ireland, Malta, Moldova, Montenegro, Poland, Russian Federation, Serbia, Slovakia, Spain (Castilla y León, Catalonia, Extremadura and Galicia), Sweden, the former Yugoslav Republic of Macedonia, United Kingdom (Scotland)

Information not available:
Bosnia and Herzegovina (Federation of Bosnia and Herzegovina and Republika Srpska), Bulgaria, Portugal, Slovenia, Spain (Murcia), Turkey, Uzbekistan

education and health sectors. The activities comprise training social skills, anti-bullying programmes, aggression replacement training and information on alcohol and substance abuse (Table 4.21, Fig. 4.4).

Many of the countries state that the main activities initiated and developed since 2005 concerning the inclusion in wider policy-making have related to adopting the topic in government action plans. In Romania, a National Programme for Mental Health has been adopted as one of the eight national public health programmes of the Ministry of Health. In Ireland, the programme A vision for change sets out the responsibilities in relation to mental health of the Health Service Executive, the Department of Health and Children and other departments.

Discussion

This chapter identified the extent to which countries have implemented policies and programmes to promote mental health, tackle stigma and discrimination and prevent mental disorders.

The findings show that interventions have been undertaken to raise awareness and to tackle stigma and discrimination in almost all countries. Many of the mental health promotion programmes focus on the general population or improving parenting and the mental health of children and adolescents, whereas the needs of the older population have only been addressed in a few countries. For the workplace, some countries have reported developments to bring the topic onto the political agenda, but few indicate concrete activities to promote mental health in this setting. Relatively many countries implemented programmes to prevent depression and suicide. Most of these activities have targeted the general population, whereas interventions that address specifically vulnerable groups have rarely been designed.

Table 4.21. Integration of mental health into the school curricula through partnership work between the education and health sectors in groups of countries

Mental health integrated into school curricula by the education and health sectors	EU		EU15		New EU countries since 2004		Israel, Norway and Switzerland		South-eastern Europe		CIS		Total	
	No.	%	No.	%	No.	%	No.	%	No.	%	No.	%	No.	%
Yes, through partnership	14	52	5	33	9	75	2	67	3	43	1	20	20	48
Yes, but not through partnership	5	19	4	27	1	8	1	33	1	14	0	0	7	17
No integration	6	22	5	33	1	8	0	0	3	43	3	60	12	29
Information not available	2	7	1	7	1	8	0	0	0	0	1	20	3	7

Fig. 4.4. Mental health is integrated into the school curricula through a partnership with the education and health sectors in countries

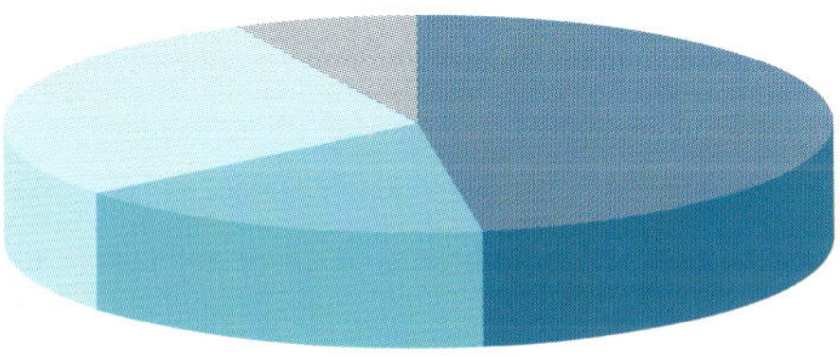

Yes, mental health is integrated into the school curricula through partnership work between the two sectors:
Belgium, Bosnia and Herzegovina (Republika Srpska), Croatia, Cyprus, Czech Republic, Denmark, Estonia, Germany, Hungary, Israel, Latvia, Lithuania, Malta, Norway, Poland, Romania, Russian Federation, Serbia, Spain (Castilla y León, Catalonia and Galicia), United Kingdom (England and Wales and Scotland)

Yes, mental health is integrated into the school curricula but not through partnership work between the two sectors:
Austria, Bosnia and Herzegovina (Federation of Bosnia and Herzegovina), Ireland, Luxembourg, Montenegro, Netherlands, Slovakia, Switzerland

No:
Albania, Azerbaijan, Bulgaria, Finland, France, Georgia, Greece, Italy, Moldova, Spain (Extremadura and Murcia), Sweden, the former Yugoslav Republic of Macedonia, Turkey

Information not available:
Portugal, Slovenia, Uzbekistan

Some of the countries comment that there have been various anti-stigma actions in the framework of the health promotion programmes, and these have been delivered in collaboration with different types of partner organizations. This shows that, although mental health promotion, anti-stigma and mental disorder prevention activities can be distinguished conceptually the strategic development of interventions in these fields overlap, and this must be kept in mind when interpreting the results of this survey.

Some countries mentioned the difficulty in obtaining funding for ongoing anti-stigma work, even though continuity in this area is an essential component for effectiveness.

In all these areas, interventions have rarely been evaluated. Evaluation can be very cost intensive. Programmes directed at the whole population need to be evaluated through large representative samples or extensive surveys, which many countries cannot afford. Target-group specific activities can be more efficient, and their evaluation provides useful information for the development of further interventions. However, the comparative effectiveness of different types of interventions and their long-term effects are not yet sufficiently known.

Many countries indicated that governments were the main funders of programmes, although nongovernmental organizations and international organizations play a major role in countries in south-eastern Europe and CIS countries. For a strong and sustained commitment to be created to invest in promoting mental health, anti-stigma work and preventing mental disorders, evidence must be produced and disseminated about which interventions are effective and efficient in both the short and long term and how to deliver them.

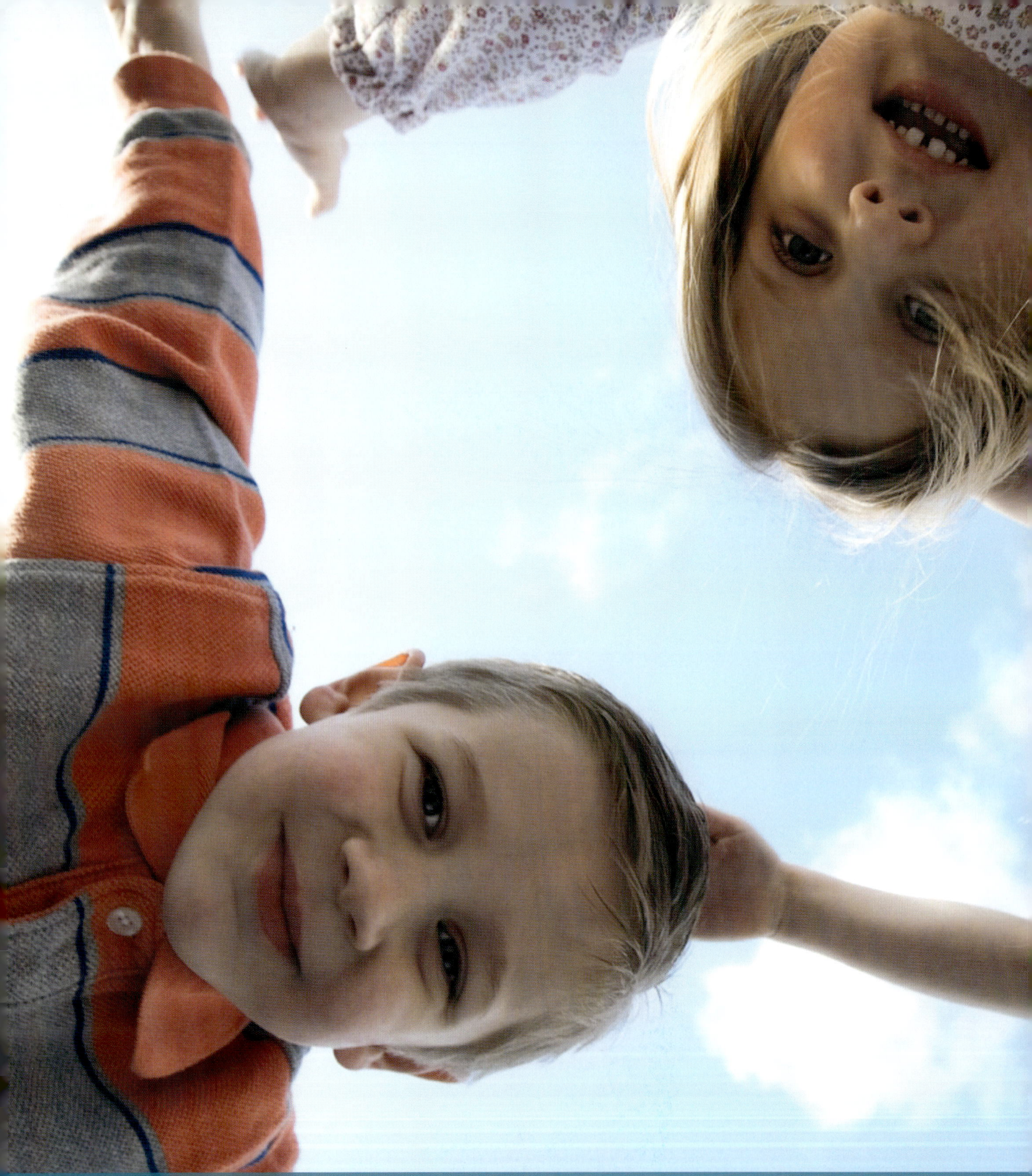

PHOTO © ANN MARIE KURTZ/I-STOCK

> *“Services in European countries appear to be so differentiated that any comparison is haphazard.”*

5. Mental health in primary care

The Mental Health Declaration for Europe strongly emphasizes the role of primary care as part of mental health services. Community-based mental health care relies on the effective functioning of primary care. This involves identifying and treating people with common mental health problems in primary care and referring people with severe mental health problems to specialist services. To achieve this, primary care has to be accessible and staffed by primary care workers who are committed and competent and have good connections with specialist services, which in turn need to offer adequate support to the primary care staff. Primary care and specialist mental health services are mutually dependent, and if either one fails the overall system fails.

The role of primary care has been underdeveloped in many parts of the European Region. In some countries, diagnosing mental disorders or prescribing psychotropic medication was (and occasionally still is) illegal for family doctors. This minimizes the motivation to detect and support people with mental disorders. This is linked to the absence of adequate training, and in combination this results in the health system marginalizing and discriminating against people with mental health problems.

This chapter investigates the state of mental health care in primary care services in European countries. The results offer some insight into the action required.

Roles of general practitioners and family doctors in mental health care

Participating countries were asked to indicate the roles of general practitioners and family doctors in mental health care that are:

- required in policy or legislation; and
- common in practice.

Roles and responsibilities were surveyed separately for people with common mental health problems (anxiety and depression) and people with severe mental health problems (bipolar disorder and schizophrenia):

- identification and referral to specialist services;
- diagnosis; and
- prescribing and treatment.

Identification and referral to specialist services

Policy or legislation specifies the roles of GPs in identifying and referring people with common and severe mental health problems in about 75% of the countries (32 of 42 countries for common disorders and 31 of 42 for severe disorders), but this takes place in about 90% of countries (Tables 5.1 and 5.2, Fig. 5.1 and 5.2).

Laws and regulation are not always the best instruments to determine roles and

Table 5.1. Roles of general practitioners and family doctors indicated in policy or legislation – identifying and referring to specialist services people with mental health problems in groups of countries

Identification and referral	EU		EU15		New EU countries since 2004		Israel, Norway and Switzerland		South-eastern Europe		CIS		Total	
	No.	%	No.	%	No.	%	No.	%	No.	%	No.	%	No.	%
Common mental health problems														
Yes	18	67	10	67	8	67	3	100	7	100	4	80	32	76
No	7	26	5	33	2	17	0	0	0	0	1	20	8	19
Information not available	2	7	0	0	2	17	0	0	0	0	0	0	2	5
Severe and enduring mental health problems														
Yes	18	67	12	80	6	50	2	67	7	100	4	80	31	74
No	5	19	3	20	2	17	1	33	0	0	1	20	7	17
Information not available	4	15	0	0	4	33	0	0	0	0	0	0	4	10

Table 5.2. Roles of general practitioners and family doctors in practice – identifying and referring to specialist services people with mental health problems in groups of countries

Identification and referral:	EU		EU15		New EU countries since 2004		Israel, Norway and Switzerland		South-eastern Europe		CIS		Total	
	No.	%	No.	%	No.	%	No.	%	No.	%	No.	%	No.	%
Common mental health problems														
Yes	25	93	15	100	10	83	3	100	7	100	5	100	40	95
Information not available	2	7	0	0	2	17	0	0	0	0	0	0	2	5
Severe and enduring mental health problems														
Yes	25	93	15	100	10	83	2	67	7	100	5	100	39	93
No	0	0	0	0	0	0	1	33	0	0	0	0	1	2
Information not available	2	7	0	0	2	17	0	0	0	0	0	0	2	5

Fig. 5.1. Roles of general practitioners and family doctors in practice – identifying and referring to specialist services people with common mental health problems in countries

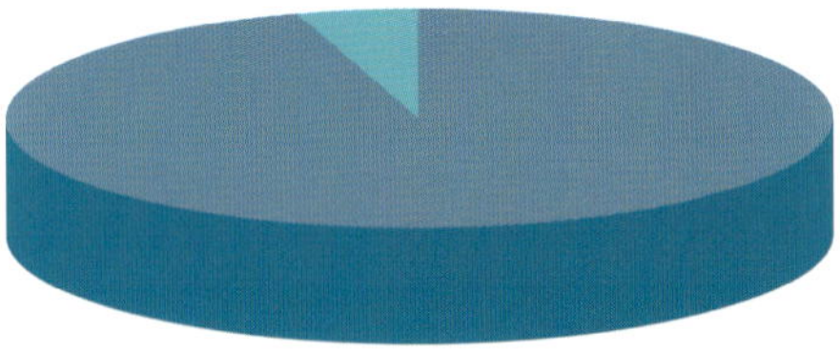

Yes:
Albania, Austria, Azerbaijan, Belgium, Bosnia and Herzegovina (Federation of Bosnia and Herzegovina and Republika Srpska), Bulgaria, Croatia, Czech Republic, Denmark, Estonia, Finland, France, Georgia, Germany, Greece, Hungary, Ireland, Israel, Italy, Latvia, Lithuania, Luxembourg, Malta, Moldova, Montenegro, Netherlands, Norway, Poland, Portugal, Romania, Russian Federation, Serbia, Slovakia, Spain (Castilla y León, Catalonia, Extremadura, Galicia and Murcia), Sweden, Switzerland, the former Yugoslav Republic of Macedonia, Turkey, United Kingdom (England and Wales and Scotland), Uzbekistan

Information not available:
Cyprus, Slovenia

Fig. 5.2. Roles of general practitioners and family doctors in practice – identifying and referring to specialist services people with severe and enduring mental health problems in countries

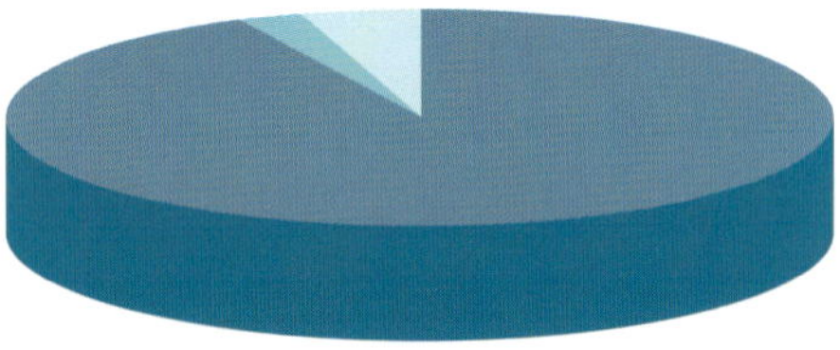

Yes:
Albania, Austria, Azerbaijan, Belgium, Bosnia and Herzegovina (Federation of Bosnia and Herzegovina and Republika Srpska), Bulgaria, Croatia, Czech Republic, Denmark, Estonia, Finland, France, Georgia, Germany, Greece, Hungary, Ireland, Italy, Latvia, Lithuania, Luxembourg, Malta, Moldova, Montenegro, Netherlands, Norway, Poland, Portugal, Romania, Russian Federation, Serbia, Slovenia, Spain (Castilla y León, Catalonia, Extremadura, Galicia and Murcia), Sweden, Switzerland, the former Yugoslav Republic of Macedonia, Turkey, United Kingdom (England and Wales and Scotland), Uzbekistan

No:
Israel

Information not available:
Cyprus, Slovakia

responsibilities that are perceived as traditional and standard practice in many countries and associated with professional ethics. In Austria, the Czech Republic, Finland, France, Greece, Hungary, Latvia, Luxembourg, the Russian Federation and Slovenia, GPs are expected to identify and refer people with common mental health problems without reference to formal regulation, and this probably applies in most other countries.

Similarly, in many countries GPs identify and refer people with severe and enduring mental disorders with or without legal requirements, as indicated by Austria, the Czech Republic, Greece, Luxembourg, Malta and the Russian Federation (no information was available for Hungary, Latvia and Slovenia).

Typical for many high-income countries is Norway: the GP has a gatekeeper function for all specialized services and refers people with a possible mental disorder to specialized services in the public sector and to psychologists and psychiatrists in private practice (for differential diagnosis and treatment).

In many countries, especially those in which mental health has only recently become part of the service package to be provided in primary care, GPs still confront challenges.

- In Latvia, GPs have difficulty recognizing mental health problems due to lack of training.
- In Lithuania, GPs are expected to treat people with common mental health problems, but a proportion of them send these people to a psychiatrist. Many people go directly to mental health centres because they believe that psychiatrists have special competence.

Diagnosis

Policies and legislation in 30 of 42 countries (71%) recognize the role of GPs in diagnosing people with common mental disorders. Significantly fewer countries (18 of 42 countries, 43%) specifically mandate GPs to diagnose people with severe and enduring mental health problems (Table 5.3).

Again, in practice, GPs in some other countries also diagnose people with common mental disorders, even when they are not formally required to do so, such as Austria, Bulgaria, the Czech Republic, France, Italy and Luxembourg. No information was available for Slovenia (Fig. 5.3).

However, 16 of 42 countries (38%) report that GPs do not diagnose severe mental disorders, and another 4 of 42 countries (10%) cannot provide information on this (Fig. 5.4). GPs diagnose severe mental disorders in 11 of the EU15 countries (73%) versus only 5 of the 12 countries that joined EU after 2004 (42%). Three of the 12 countries that joined EU after 2004 (25%) cannot provide information on whether GPs undertake this role or not (Table 5.4).

All the countries in south-eastern Europe indicate that GPs diagnose people with common mental health problems, but they only diagnose severe mental disorders in Croatia, Montenegro and Serbia.

Of the CIS countries participating in this survey, GPs in the Russian Federation and Uzbekistan diagnose common mental health problems. Uzbekistan also reports that GPs diagnose severe mental disorders, but this is just a preliminary diagnosis that does not affect the social rights of the people with mental disorders (for example, benefit claims cannot be made based on this diagnosis).

Current practices in some countries include the following.

Table 5.3. Roles of general practitioners and family doctors as indicated in policy or legislation – diagnosing people with mental health problems in groups of countries

	EU		EU15		New EU countries since 2004		Israel, Norway and Switzerland		South-eastern Europe		CIS		Total	
Diagnosis	No	%	No	%	No.	%	No.	%	No.	%	No.	%	No.	%
Common mental health problems														
Yes	10	67	10	67	8	67	3	100	7	100	2	40	30	71
No	6	22	4	27	2	17	0	0	0	0	3	60	9	21
Information not available	3	11	1	7	2	17	0	0	0	0	0	0	3	7
Severe and enduring mental health problems														
Yes	11	41	7	47	4	33	1	33	4	57	2	40	18	43
No	9	33	7	47	2	17	1	33	3	43	3	60	16	38
Information not available	7	26	1	7	6	50	1	33	0	0	0	0	8	19

Fig. 5.3. Roles of general practitioners and family doctors in practice – diagnosing people with common mental health problems in countries

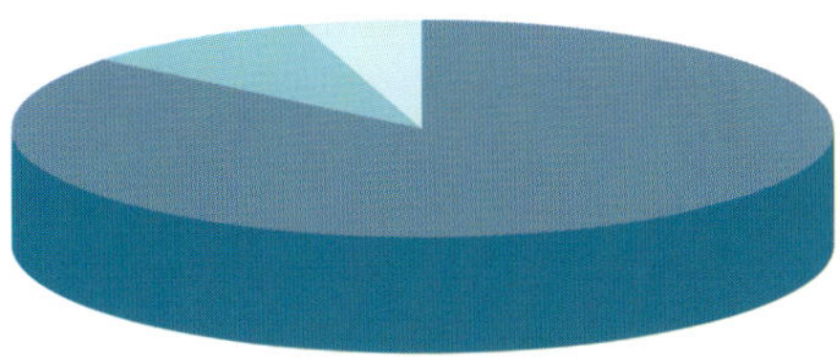

Yes: Albania, Austria, Belgium, Bosnia and Herzegovina (Federation of Bosnia and Herzegovina and Republika Srpska), Bulgaria, Croatia, Czech Republic, Denmark, Estonia, Finland, France, Germany, Ireland, Israel, Italy, Latvia, Lithuania, Luxembourg, Malta, Montenegro, Netherlands, Norway, Poland, Portugal, Romania, Russian Federation, Serbia, Slovakia, Slovenia, Spain (Castilla y León, Catalonia, Extremadura, Galicia, Murcia), Sweden, Switzerland, the former Yugoslav Republic of Macedonia, Turkey, United Kingdom (England and Wales and Scotland), Uzbekistan

No:
Azerbaijan, Georgia, Hungary, Moldova

Information not available:
Cyprus, Greece

Fig. 5.4. Roles of general practitioners and family doctors in practice – diagnosing people with severe and enduring mental health problems in countries

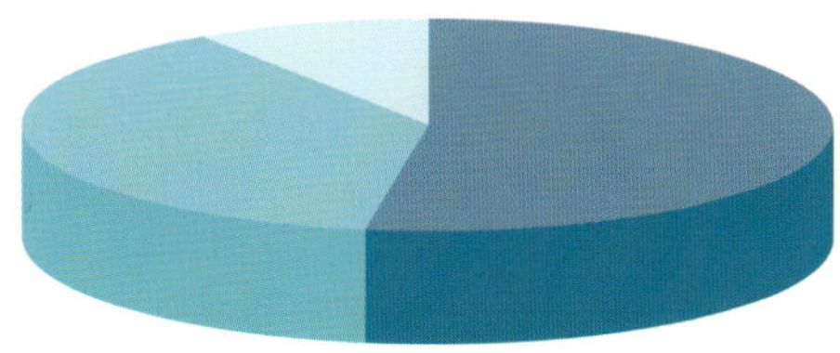

Yes:
Austria, Belgium, Bulgaria, Croatia, Cyprus, Denmark, Estonia, France, Germany, Ireland, Lithuania, Luxembourg, Montenegro, Netherlands, Norway, Poland, Serbia, Spain (Castilla y León, Catalonia, Extremadura, Galicia and Murcia), Sweden, Switzerland, United Kingdom (England and Wales and Scotland), Uzbekistan

No:
Albania, Azerbaijan, Bosnia and Herzegovina (Federation of Bosnia and Herzegovina and Republika Srpska), Czech Republic, Finland, Georgia, Hungary, Israel, Italy, Latvia, Moldova, Portugal, Romania, Russian Federation, the former Yugoslav Republic of Macedonia, Turkey

Information not available:
Greece, Malta, Slovakia, Slovenia

Table 5.4. Roles of general practitioners and family doctors in practice – diagnosing people with mental health problems in groups of countries

Diagnosis	EU		EU15		New EU countries since 2004		Israel, Norway and Switzerland		South-eastern Europe		CIS		Total	
	No.	%	No.	%	No.	%	No.	%	No.	%	No.	%	No.	%
Common mental health problems														
Yes	24	89	14	93	10	83	3	100	7	100	2	40	36	86
No	1	4	0	0	1	8	0	0	0	0	3	60	4	10
Information not available	2	7	1	7	1	8	0	0	0	0	0	0	2	5
Severe and enduring mental health problems														
Yes	16	59	11	73	5	42	2	67	3	43	1	20	22	52
No	7	26	3	20	4	33	1	33	4	57	4	80	16	38
Information not available	4	15	1	7	3	25	0	0	0	0	0	0	4	10

- In Belgium, for diagnosing severe problems, GPs may refer people to specialized mental health services.
- In the United Kingdom (Scotland), specialists usually confirm the diagnosis of severe and enduring mental health problems, unlike common mental health problems, which primary care mainly diagnoses.

The process of making a diagnosis can have important implications that vary from country to country; a formal diagnosis of a mental health condition may allow the individual to access particular services or benefits or can have negative social and employment effects. The mandate and competence therefore have to be related to the specific rules in each country.

Treatment

In most of the countries where GPs are assigned (by policy or legislation) to diagnose common mental health problems they are also assigned to treat them. GPs in 36 of 42 countries (86%) regularly treat people with common disorders, including in countries where policy or legislation do not specify this (Tables 5.5 and 5.6, Fig. 5.5).

Treatment of severe disorders is the least acknowledged role of GPs across the European countries. The policies and legislation of 14 of 42 countries (33%) include this role, and GPs practise this role in 17 of 42 countries (40%). In addition to 13 of the EU15 countries, Norway and Switzerland, only Cyprus and Malta of the countries that joined the EU after 2004 report that GPs undertake this role regularly (Fig. 5.6).

In 8 of the 21 countries where GPs treat people with severe mental disorders, this is based on tradition and professional ethics rather than policy or legislative requirements (Austria, France, Greece, Luxembourg, Malta, Netherlands, Sweden and Switzerland have no requirements).

In contrast, in countries such as Bulgaria, Latvia, Romania, the former Yugoslav Republic of Macedonia and Uzbekistan, policies or legislation request that GPs take an active role in treating people with severe mental disorders, but this is not yet common practice.

Current practices include the following.

- In Belgium, GPs are expected to refer people with severe mental health problems to specialized mental health services for treatment. However, doctors are autonomous in their treatment decisions, so this is merely a guideline and not a binding rule.
- In Denmark, severe and enduring mental problems are usually treated only in collaboration with or supervised by community and hospital psychiatric services.
- In Poland, GPs treat people with common mental health problems pharmaceutically but do not use psychotherapy.
- In Spain (Murcia), GPs collaborate in treating and following up people with severe disorders, but the responsibility remains with the mental health specialists.

Fig. 5.5. Roles of general practitioners and family doctors in practice – treating people with common mental health problems in countries

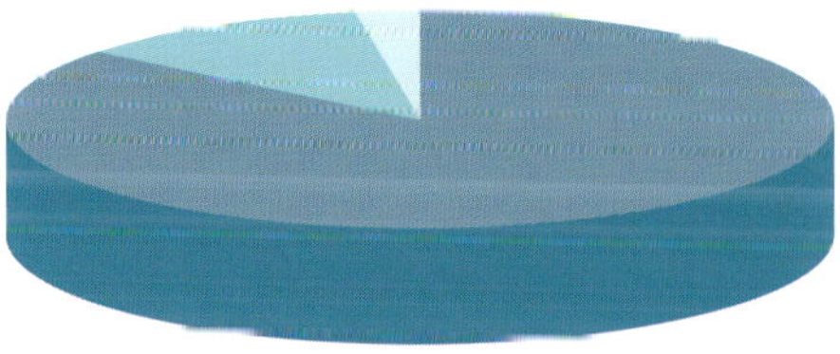

Yes:
Albania, Austria, Belgium, Bosnia and Herzegovina (Federation of Bosnia and Herzegovina and Republika Srpska), Bulgaria, Croatia, Denmark, Estonia, Finland, France, Germany, Greece, Hungary, Ireland, Israel, Italy, Latvia, Lithuania, Luxembourg, Malta, Moldova, Montenegro, Netherlands, Norway, Poland, Portugal, Romania, Russian Federation, Serbia, Slovakia, Slovenia, Spain (Castilla y León, Catalonia, Extremadura, Galicia and Murcia), Sweden, Switzerland, Turkey, United Kingdom (England and Wales and Scotland)

No:
Azerbaijan, Czech Republic, Georgia, the former Yugoslav Republic of Macedonia, Uzbekistan

Information not available:
Cyprus

Fig. 5.6. Roles of general practitioners and family doctors in practice – treating people with severe and enduring mental health problems in countries

Yes:
Austria, Belgium, Cyprus, Denmark, Finland, France, Germany, Greece, Ireland, Luxembourg, Malta, Netherlands, Norway, Spain (Catalonia, Extremadura, Galicia, Murcia), Sweden, Switzerland, United Kingdom (England and Wales and Scotland)

No:
Albania, Azerbaijan, Bosnia and Herzegovina (Federation of Bosnia and Herzegovina), Bosnia and Herzegovina (Republika Srpska), Bulgaria, Croatia, Czech Republic, Georgia, Hungary, Israel, Italy, Latvia, Moldova, Montenegro, Portugal, Romania, Russian Federation, Serbia, Spain (Castilla y León), the former Yugoslav Republic of Macedonia, Turkey, Uzbekistan

Information not available:
Estonia, Lithuania, Poland, Slovakia, Slovenia

Table 5.5. Roles of general practitioners and family doctors indicated in policy or legislation – treating people with mental health problems in groups of countries

Treatment	EU		EU15		New EU countries since 2004		Israel, Norway and Switzerland		South-eastern Europe		CIS		Total	
	No.	%	No.	%	No.	%	No.	%	No.	%	No.	%	No.	%
Common mental health problems														
Yes	19	70	10	67	9	75	3	100	6	86	2	40	30	71
No	6	22	5	33	1	8	0	0	1	14	3	60	10	24
Information not available	2	7	0	0	2	17	0	0	0	0	0	0	2	5
Severe and enduring mental health problems														
Yes	10	37	7	47	3	25	0	0	3	43	1	20	14	33
No	11	41	8	53	3	25	2	67	4	57	4	80	21	50
Information not available	6	22	0	0	6	50	1	33	0	0	0	0	7	17

Table 5.6. Roles of general practitioners and family doctors in practice – treating people with mental health problems in groups of countries

Treatment	EU		EU15		New EU countries since 2004		Israel, Norway and Switzerland		South-eastern Europe		CIS		Total	
	No.	%	No.	%	No.	%	No.	%	No.	%	No.	%	No.	%
Common mental health problems														
Yes	25	93	15	100	10	83	3	100	6	86	2	40	36	86
No	1	4	0	0	1	8	0	0	1	14	3	60	5	12
Information not available	1	4	0	0	1	8	0	0	0	0	0	0	1	2
Severe and enduring mental health problems														
Yes	15	56	13	87	2	17	2	67	0	0	0	0	17	40
No	7	26	2	13	5	42	1	33	7	100	5	100	20	48
Information not available	5	19	0	0	5	42	0	0	0	0	0	0	5	12

Challenges for GPs who treat people with mental health problems include the following.

- In Georgia, family doctors have not received relevant education to treat people with mental health problems.
- In Latvia, GPs have great difficulty in providing treatment for people with mental health problems and mostly use tranquillizers.
- In Norway, psychological and psychiatric issues are not very prominent in the education of the GPs, but they are expected to provide services for people with common mental health problems.

When policy or legislation requires GPs to treat people with mental health problems, this can imply that the treatment offered will be an isolated mental health intervention. The physical health and social needs risk being ignored. Primary care staff members are responsible for the physical health needs of those with common or severe mental disorders in all countries.

Limitations on the role of general practitioners and family doctors in treating people with mental disorders

Of the 42 countries, 31 (74%) set limits on the treatment GPs can provide for people with mental disorders (Table 5.7). These limitations fall into several categories.

Right to prescribe medication

- In the Czech Republic, Estonia, Slovakia and Slovenia, GPs are not allowed to prescribe some new types of psychotropic medication.

- In Denmark, legislation and guidelines from the National Board of Health set some limitations on prescribing of drugs etc., especially for children and adolescents.
- In Israel, GPs and family doctors can only prescribe antipsychotic medication in consultation with a psychiatrist.
- In Romania, GPs can prescribe antidepressants only as indicated by a psychiatrist.
- In the Russian Federation, GPs cannot prescribe medication such as some benzodiazepines.
- In Spain (Galicia) and Finland, GPs cannot prescribe clozapine.

Right to perform certain tasks

- In Albania, family doctors cannot initiate treatment without a recommendation from the specialized service.
- In Croatia, GPs cannot provide treatment for people with severe and enduring mental health problems.
- In Georgia, the state certificate enables the family doctors to diagnose and treat only some common conditions. However, since the training is very brief, family doctors do not obtain adequate knowledge and only diagnose and treat with the back-up of psychiatrists.
- In Germany, special qualifications are required to meet existing guidelines for certain types of treatment. These include psychotherapy, the prescription of ambulant psychiatric health care and sociotherapy.
- In Switzerland, family doctors and psychiatrists have the same rights with respect to therapy (such as prescription of medicines, referral to psychotherapy and hospitalization in clinics) and legal measures (such as involuntary admission). Certain differences related to the funding of psychotherapeutic services depend on the relevant qualifications.
- In the United Kingdom (England and Wales), the standards of the National Service Framework for Mental Health outline the role of primary care in mental health, and the National Institute for Clinical Excellence publishes national guidelines for clinical practice, such as guidelines for schizophrenia and depression, but these are not mandatory.

Pressure on mental health care in primary care

- In Austria, there is a limited time frame in primary care; near zero remuneration for mental health interventions (such as counselling); psychotherapeutic interventions by primary care physicians are practically not available for reimbursement by national health plans; primary care physicians cannot perform procedures that are restricted to hospital-based mental health care.
- In the Netherlands, GPs experience too little time and too high workload; for some mental disorders GPs lack knowledge about treatment.
- In Poland, there are no limitations but there are obstacles in practice concerning the knowledge of GPs on mental health problems and psychotherapy.

Table 5.7. Limitations on what general practitioners and family doctors can do related to treating people with mental disorders in groups of countries

Limitations	EU		EU15		New EU countries since 2004		Israel, Norway and Switzerland		South-eastern Europe		CIS		Total	
	No.	%	No.	%	No.	%	No.	%	No.	%	No.	%	No.	%
Yes	19	70	11	73	8	67	3	100	5	71	4	80	31	74
No	8	30	4	27	4	33	0	0	2	29	1	20	11	26

Availability of national guidelines on assessment and treatment for GPs dealing with people with mental health problems

Countries were asked to indicate whether national assessment and treatment guidelines are available for key mental health conditions in general practices and family practices (Tables 5.8). They were asked to specify whether the guidelines addressed common or severe mental disorders.

Almost 70% of countries have some type of treatment guidelines for key mental health conditions in general practices, especially the EU15 countries (80%) and Israel, Norway and Switzerland. Family medicine is relatively new in many countries in the eastern part of the Region, but about 50% of the countries that joined the EU after 2004, 71% of the countries in south-eastern Europe and 40% of the CIS countries also indicate that they have such guidelines for GPs.

Guidelines are valuable in ensuring that clinicians provide high-quality up-to-date evidence-based care and that the public and users of services know what standards of care should be offered. The challenge is that, whereas developing and publishing guidelines is relatively straightforward, ensuring that clinicians comply with those guidelines is much harder.

Guidelines from European countries include the following.

- Finland: current care practice guidelines are available for schizophrenia, depression, alcohol problems, substance abuse problems, eating disorders of children and adolescents and nicotine dependence.
- Germany:
  - Since 1995, the Association of the Scientific Medical Societies in Germany has been coordinating the development of guidelines for diagnosis and therapy, at the request of the Advisory Council on the Assessment of Developments in the Health Care System, through individual scientific and medical societies.
  - The Federal Joint Committee is responsible for an independent German Institute for Quality and Efficiency in Health Care. The Institute deals with issues that are important for the quality and efficiency of services within statutory health insurance, especially in the following areas:
    1. research, presentation and assessment of current medical knowledge related to diagnostic and therapeutic procedures in selected illnesses;
    2. compiling scientific papers, expert opinions and position papers on questions related to the quality and efficiency of services;
    3. assessing evidence-based guidelines for the most important epidemiological illnesses;
    4. submitting recommendations on disease management programmes;

Table 5.8. Availability of national guidelines on assessment and treatment of key mental health conditions for general practitioners and family doctors in groups of countries

National guidelines	EU		EU15		New EU countries since 2004		Israel, Norway and Switzerland		South-eastern Europe		CIS		Total	
	No.	%	No.	%	No.	%	No.	%	No.	%	No.	%	No.	%
Yes	18	67	12	80	6	50	3	100	5	71	2	40	28	67
Common mental disorders	9	34	6	40	3	25	2	67	1	14	1	20	13	31
Severe and enduring mental disorders	3	11	1	7	2	17	0	0	1	14	0	0	4	10
Both	6	22	5	33	1	8	1	33	3	43	1	20	11	26
No	9	33	3	20	6	50	0	0	2	29	3	60	14	33

5. assessing the effectiveness of medication; and
6. preparing information on the quality and efficiency of health care understandable to all citizens.

- The Federal Joint Committee is the supreme decision-making body of Germany's health care system. The Committee includes representatives of physicians, dentists, hospitals, sickness funds and patients. The Committee passes the guidelines necessary to ensure the provision of sufficient, rational and economical care for insured parties; in this context, special requirements with regard to care for people who are disabled or are in danger of becoming disabled and people who are mentally ill must be considered.
- Hungary: guidelines about specific disorders include paragraphs or references for GPs. No psychiatric guidelines designed for GPs have been published.

Refresher training courses in the rational use of psychotropic drugs and in psychosocial intervention

Countries were asked to provide information about refresher training courses for family doctors and to specify the proportion of primary health care doctors with at least two days of training in the past year in the rational use of psychotropic drugs and in psychosocial (non-biological) interventions.

Data are not available for about 80% of countries. Only 10 countries provided information on training courses in psychotropic drugs and 9 countries on training courses in psychosocial interventions, but this information is highly speculative. Only in Germany have 100% of family doctors received retraining, since this is obligatory. Serbia reported that 60% were trained in psychotropic drug prescribing, since the Institute of Mental Health trains GPs continually.

Many countries indicate that courses are available but that no reliable data are available on the number of participants. This might be due to the variety of activities that account for refresher training in countries, such as:

- presentations of new drugs organized and conducted by pharmaceutical companies;
- professional conferences where GPs participate; and
- retraining of physicians who were recently reassigned as family doctors after primary care medicine was reorganized in CIS countries.

There were a few comments from countries for which information is not available.

- Austria: participation in refreshers is up to doctors. Continuing medical education is compulsory for all licensed doctors, but there are no penalties if doctors do not renew their continuing medical education certificates. Several continuing medical education interventions are offered in the Austrian continuing medical education calendar.
- Bulgaria: there are a number of training courses and study tours under a variety of foreign-sponsored programmes and projects such as the Phare project of the European Commission, the South-eastern Europe Mental Health Project (Enhancing Social Cohesion through Strengthening Community Mental Health Services in South-eastern Europe), bilateral collaboration with Belgium (the Flemish Region) etc. The information for these training events is not collected and aggregated at the national level.
- Latvia, Moldova and the former Yugoslav Republic of Macedonia indicate that, although there might be some occasional training, no training courses for GPs are organized regularly.
- Serbia has regular courses for GPs. In addition, Serbia and Bosnia and Herzegovina collaborate on continuing medical education for GPs, supported by the Norwegian Medical Association. Joint annual programmes on mental health issues in general practice are organized in both countries with the same curricula. The project includes evaluation. Study tours are also organized for GPs in both countries.

Main activities initiated and developed since 2005 related to mental health services in primary health care

Many examples were given of activities initiated since January 2005.

Training

- Austria: a research project on mental health in general practice, which will include psychiatry in the training of general practitioners.
- Germany: additional training within the framework of care focusing on family doctors. The introduction of a system of care focusing on family doctors introduced by the Health System Modernization Act of 2004 also increases doctors' obligations to participate in ongoing training. Mental health plays an essential role in this context.
- Russian Federation: the courses on psychiatry were added to the system of professional postgraduate education of GPs. A project establishing protocols on disease management and standards of providing medical care in psychiatry, which started in 2005, is ending.
- United Kingdom (England and Wales): in 2007, the government announced £170 million in additional funding over three years to establish services and training to improve access to evidence-based psychological therapy focused on anxiety and depression currently dealt with in primary care with access to specialist support. The approach is outlined in national guidelines published by the National Institute for Clinical Excellence.
- Uzbekistan: the Ministry of Health and WHO developed and published a manual on mental health protection in primary health care in Uzbekistan.

Structural changes

- Finland: "depression nurses" were introduced in primary care.
- Georgia: the number of trained family doctors has increased significantly (in 2004 there were 100 and now there are 1500).
- United Kingdom (England and Wales): a Primary Care Development Unit is planned that will fulfil the role of a centre of excellence for primary care outlined in a WHO position paper[1]. Further development is planned for the incentive payments for GPs delivering mental health care.

Discussion

The results of this survey inform about the role of GPs and primary care services in mental health care in the European Region. Whereas roles and responsibilities are quite consistent and wide-ranging for common mental disorders, they are more varied and limited in the care of people with severe mental disorders.

For common mental health problems, most national mental health policies expect GPs to identify, diagnose, refer and treat. For severe mental disorders, GPs are again mandated to play a major role in identifying, diagnosing and referring people, but treatment in most countries is expected to be the responsibility of specialists, with GPs playing a supportive role. This applies particularly to CIS countries.

Intriguingly, except for the treatment of severe mental disorders, the role of family doctors seems to extend beyond the responsibilities that are specified in policy guidance in several countries. This is probably explained by a combination of tradition, expectations, commitment, ethics and common sense. Minor self-limiting conditions do not require referral to pressured specialists.

GPs in the EU15 countries, Israel, Norway and Switzerland are also very involved in treating severe mental disorders. In contrast, only a minority of the countries joining the EU since 2004, countries in south-eastern Europe and CIS countries report a role for their GPs in practice, slightly lower than permitted by policies. There may be a few important reasons for this, with ramifications for the functioning of the mental health system.

1 Cohen A. *Position paper – primary care mental health in Europe*. Copenhagen, WHO Regional Office for Europe, 2007.

First, GPs in much of the eastern part of the European Region are actively discouraged, sometimes even by legislation, from becoming involved with mental disorders. Mental health education is absent, and people with mental health problems distrust their competence. Second, mental health services do not have the capacity to offer support, partly because people access specialist services directly. Third, the structure of primary care in these countries is not generic but staffed by such specialists as obstetricians, paediatricians and internists, who are not inclined to address mental disorders.

After 1990, inspired by the Declaration of Alma-Ata on primary care, countries instigated reforms of primary care, including comprehensive retraining of specialists into generalists. However, the mental health component was not perceived as a priority at that time, and countries are now aiming to remedy this, influenced by the realization of the very high burden of disease attributable to mental disorders. A concern is the lack of systematic retraining, as this survey identified.

This survey did not consider the variation in the structure and funding of primary care. In many European countries, GPs operate as single practitioners. In some western European countries they are supported by a team of variable size, but specialist mental health staff members are included in the primary care team in very few countries (England and Finland). This and reimbursement systems have obvious implications for the capacity of primary care to offer interventions, particularly those of a social nature.

Primary care and specialist services are highly interdependent. If GPs increased their referral rate, specialist services would be unable to cope with demand. Improving the skills of primary care staff and improving the provision of services in primary care – one challenge identified by the Mental Health Declaration for Europe – requires not only changing the structure and functioning of primary care but changing how specialist services function as well. In many countries, mental health services are not set up yet to support primary care, causing suffering and inefficiency since this results in both a lack of identification of mental health needs and a large number of unnecessary referrals.

A frequent comment is the need for GPs to recognize the mental health problems behind the presentation of physical symptoms. Equally important is avoiding the neglect of physical problems of people presenting with mental disorders. There are well-known associations between mental disorders and several long-term conditions such as diabetes, ischaemic heart disease and chronic obstructive pulmonary disease, in some cases as side effects of psychotropic medication. In the countries where specialist teams have sole responsibility for the care of people with severe mental disorders, ensuring that GPs address their physical health is important. This requires active cooperation between the tiers of care. In some cases this can be supported by guidelines, but it needs to be underpinned by a shared understanding of the roles and responsibilities of the professionals involved in the care of the individual.

In common across the large majority of countries in the European Region is the absence of regulation of continuing education for primary care despite the changes in structure and roles. Continuing education seems to be open to any supplier willing to invest. This is of concern considering the comprehensive changes in role and competencies that are required from primary care if mental health reforms are to be effective.

Finally, many countries report producing treatment guidelines for primary care, especially for common mental health problems. Comparing such guidelines would be instructive. Either consistency would suggest duplication of effort or inconsistency would raise concern about differences in evidence-based care across the Region. No one can answer this question currently.

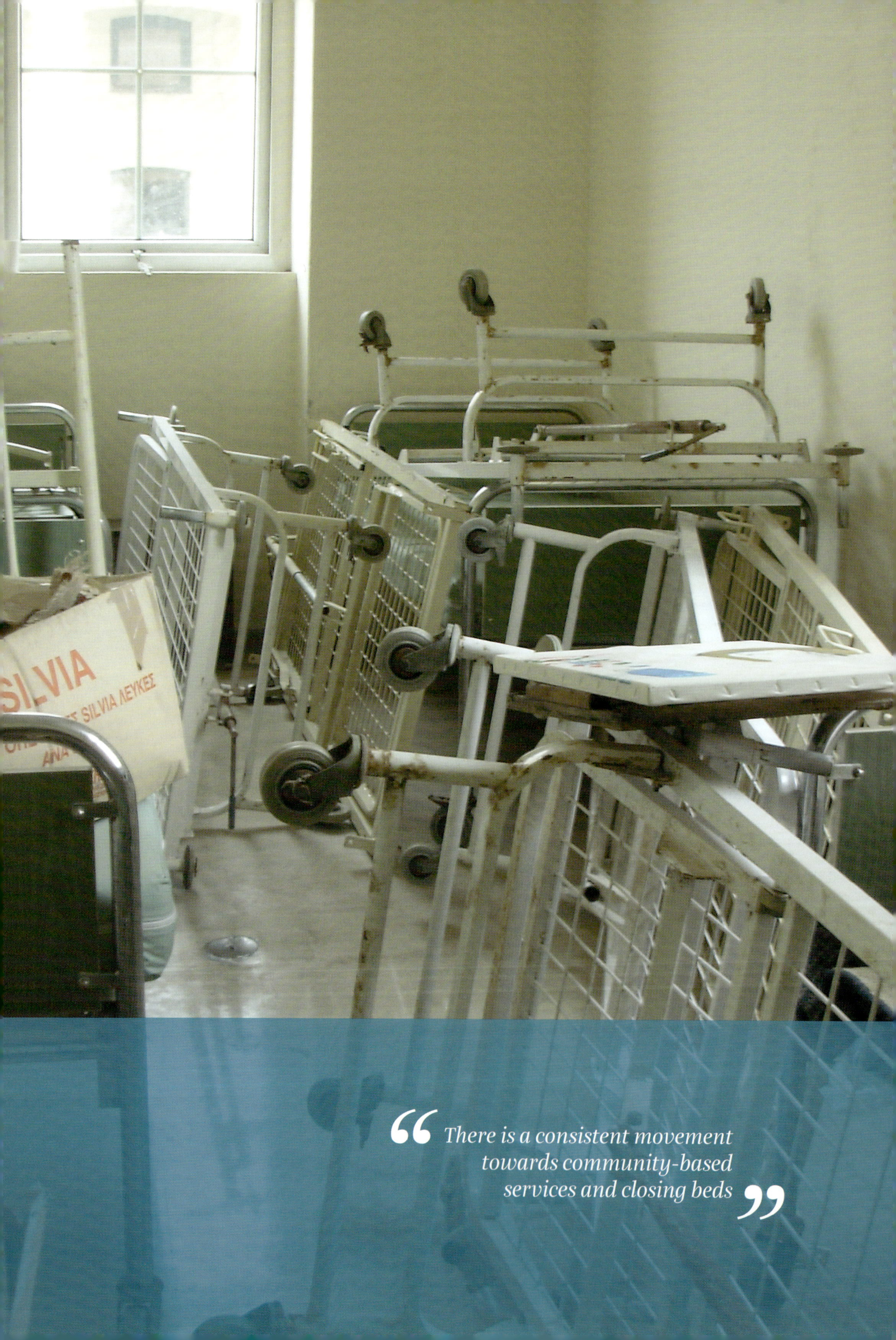

“There is a consistent movement towards community-based services and closing beds”

6. Mental health services

This chapter offers information on specialist mental health services, ranging from mental hospitals to specialist community teams, and covers services for all age groups, including children and older people. These services are the heart of mental health care, accounting for the vast majority of expenditure. However, investment patterns may differ considerably across the components of the services.

The chapter also includes access to psychosocial interventions and prescribing patterns. Finally, it looks at the availability of services for language and ethnic minority groups.

The data would be expected to vary greatly across the WHO European Region for every variable according to differences in service structure, economic status and the priority given to mental health care in countries.

Inpatient services

Availability of specialized mental health facilities

Mental hospitals

Mental hospitals are available in all countries except Italy. However, this study does not provide information about the structure and quality of mental hospitals. In some countries mental hospitals are still large institutions, but in some countries in western Europe, mental hospitals can mean purpose-built, stand-alone and relatively small-scale units close to communities.

- Bulgaria: the existing facilities are established unequally around the country, and the number of people served therefore varies.
- Finland: high variation in population coverage, from 26 200 to 560 905 inhabitants per hospital.
- Latvia: Latvia has six mental hospitals for adults: four regional ones and two for people with chronic mental disorders.
- Norway: varies substantially: from 23 000 to 100 000 inhabitants per hospital.

Definition

This survey defined a mental hospital as a specialized hospital-based facility that provides inpatient care and long-stay residential services for people with mental disorders. Usually these facilities are independent and stand-alone, although they may be linked with the rest of the health care system. The level of specialization varies considerably: in some cases only long-stay custodial services are offered, and in others specialized and short-term services are also available, such as rehabilitation services and specialist units for children and older people.

Mental hospitals include both public and private not-for-profit and for-profit facilities; mental hospitals solely for children and adolescents and mental hospitals for other specific groups (such as older people) are also included.

Mental hospitals exclude community-based psychiatric inpatient units, forensic inpatient units and forensic hospitals as well as facilities that solely treat people with alcohol and substance abuse disorder or mental retardation without an accompanying diagnosis of mental disorder.

Community-based psychiatric inpatient units and units in district general hospitals

Community-based psychiatric inpatient units and psychiatric beds in district general hospitals are available in all countries except Azerbaijan, Georgia, Moldova and Montenegro.

In most countries they refer only to psychiatric units in district general hospitals.

- Czech Republic: 32 psychiatric departments in general hospitals.
- Slovakia: no community-based units, only units within general hospitals.

In some countries that report psychiatric beds in the community in addition to district general hospitals, they refer to beds in dispensaries.

- Bulgaria: many of the outpatient community-based services (dispensaries) have become inpatient wards with variable numbers of beds (from 40 to 150).

Beds in inpatient facilities

Beds per 100 000 population

The combined rate of psychiatric beds per 100 000 population in community psychiatric inpatient units, units in district general hospitals and mental hospitals ranges from 185 in Malta to 8 in Italy, with a median rate of 72 (Table 6.1, Fig. 6.1). The variation across countries reflects differences in both the organization of mental health services and investment, as indicated by the fact that Italy and the United Kingdom (England and Wales) have rates similar to those of Albania and Turkey. In Italy and the United Kingdom (England and Wales), having few beds indicates post-deinstitutionalization, whereas having few beds in Albania and Turkey indicates low investment and the absence of service infrastructure.

Fig. 6.1. Total beds per 100 000 population in community psychiatric inpatient units and units in district general hospitals and mental hospitals in countries

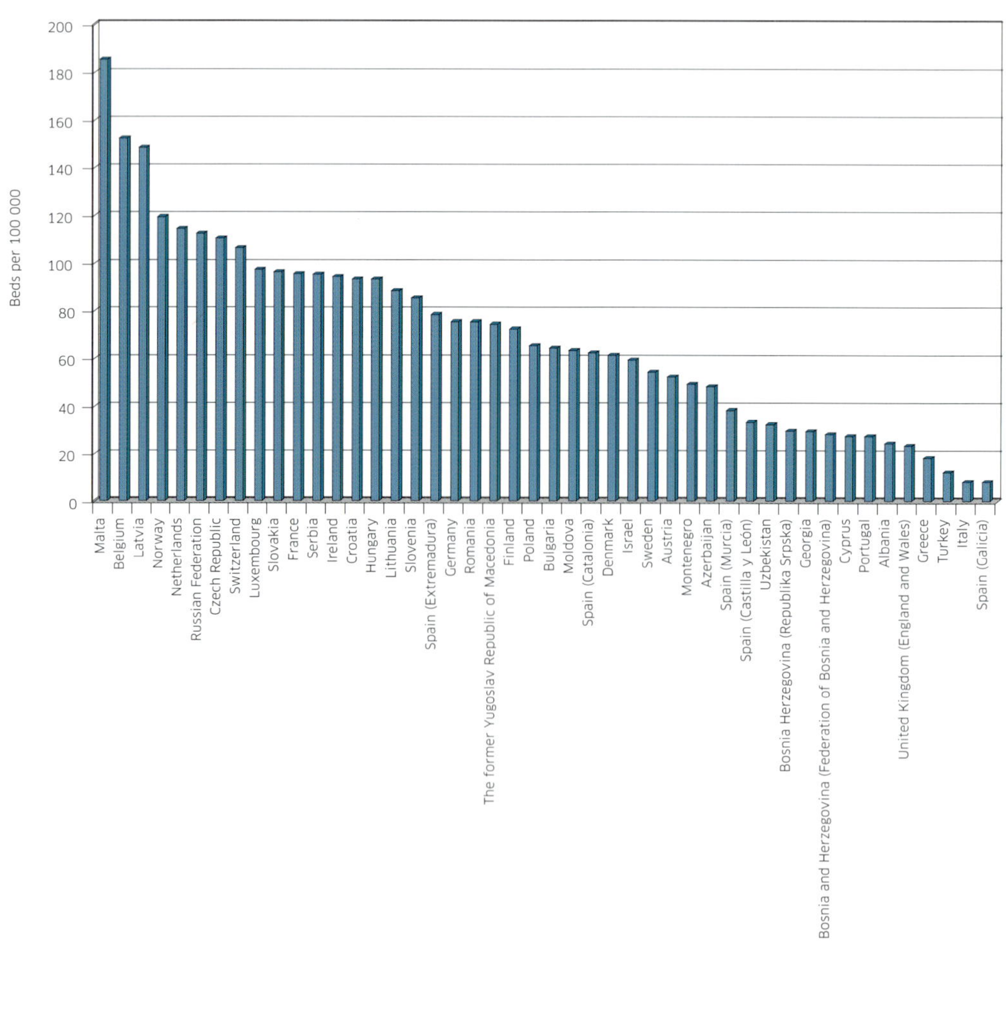

Table 6.1. Total number of beds per 100 000 population and distribution in countries

Country	Beds per 100 000 population		
	Total	Mental hospitals	Community psychiatric inpatient units and units in district general hospitals
Albania	24	18	6
Austria	52	37	15
Azerbaijan	48	48	0
Belgium	152	152	Information not available
Bosnia and Herzegovina			
Federation of Bosnia and Herzegovina	27.8	Information not available	Information not available
Republika Srpska	29.3	21.5	7.8
Bulgaria	64	28	36
Croatia	93	Information not available	Information not available
Cyprus	27	21	6
Czech Republic	110	96	14
Denmark	61	Information not available	Information not available
Estonia	Information not available	Information not available	Information not available
Finland	72	Information not available	Information not available
France	95.2	Information not available	Information not available
Georgia	29	29	0
Germany	75	Information not available	Information not available
Greece	18	14	4
Hungary	93	Information not available	Information not available
Ireland	94	71	23
Israel	59	55	4
Italy	8	0	8
Latvia	148	137	11
Lithuania	88	78	10
Luxembourg	97	52	45
Malta	185	185	0
Moldova	63	63	0
Montenegro	49	49	0
Netherlands	114	Information not available	Information not available
Norway	119	69	50
Poland	65	49	16
Portugal	27	17	10
Romania	75	54	21
Russian Federation	112	Information not available	Information not available
Serbia	95	Information not available	Information not available
Slovakia	96	18	78
Slovenia	85	72	13
Spain			
Castilla y Léon	33	23	10
Catalonia	62	46	16
Extremadura	78	73	5
Galicia	8	0	8
Murcia	38	31	7
Sweden	54	4	50
Switzerland	106	100	6
The former Yugoslav Republic of Macedonia	74	64	10
Turkey	12	9	3
United Kingdom			
England and Wales	23	14	9
Scotland	Information not available	Information not available	Information not available
Uzbekistan	32	31	1

Definition

A community-based psychiatric inpatient unit has been defined as a psychiatric unit that provides inpatient care for the management of mental disorders within a community-based facility. These units are usually located within general hospitals, but sometimes some beds are provided as part of a community centre. Community-based beds mostly provide care to users with acute problems, and the period of stay is usually short (weeks to months).

This category includes: both public and private not-for-profit and for-profit facilities; community-based psychiatric inpatient units for children and adolescents only; and community-based psychiatric inpatient units for other specific groups (such as older people).

This category excludes: mental hospitals; community residential facilities; and facilities that solely treat people with alcohol and substance abuse disorder or mental retardation or developmental disability.

Fig. 6.2. Distribution of beds per 100 000 population in mental hospitals and in community psychiatric inpatient units and units in district general hospitals in countries

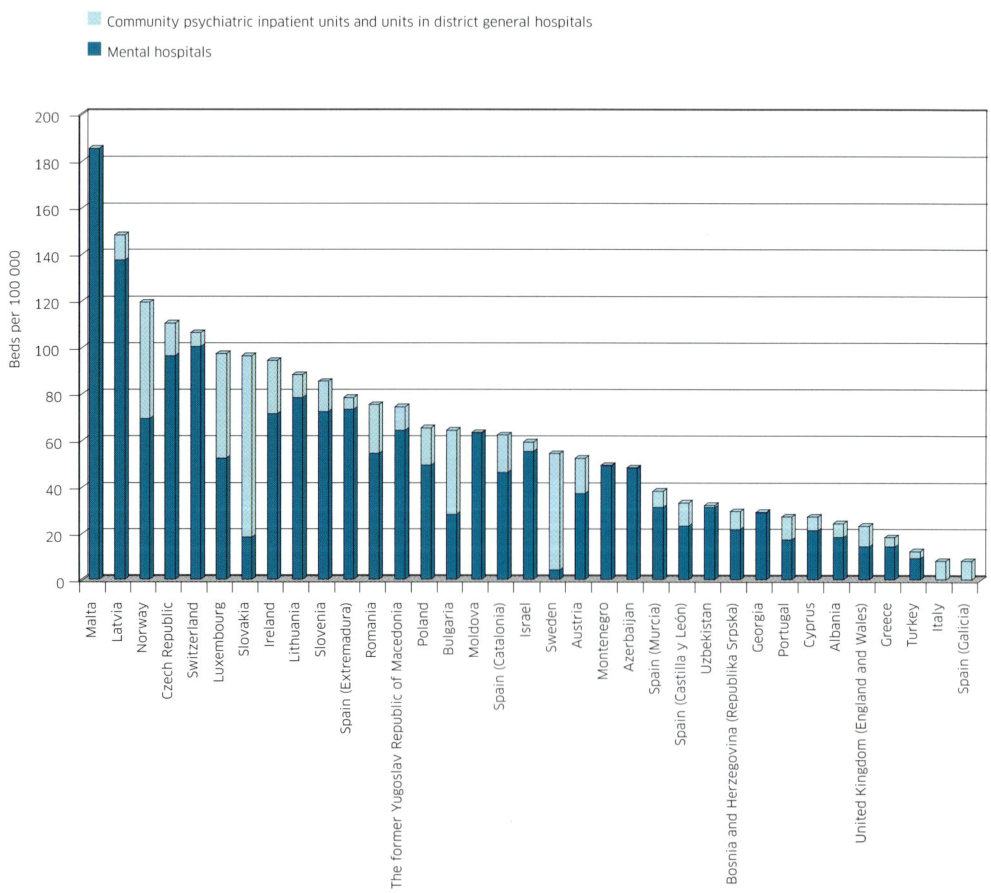

Distribution of beds by mental hospitals and community psychiatric inpatient units and units in district general hospitals

Data on the distribution of psychiatric beds in community psychiatric inpatient units and units in district general hospitals versus mental hospitals are available for some countries (Table 6.1, Fig. 6.2). In countries where information is available, most beds are in mental hospitals, except for Italy (with no mental hospitals), Slovakia and Sweden.

Median number of days in the facility

Twenty-six countries provided information on the median number of days spent in mental hospitals and community-based psychiatric inpatient units (Table 6.2). Community-based beds are invariably used for brief admissions, whereas mental hospital beds can be used for short- or long-stay admissions or for mixed purposes.

Admissions to inpatient units

Rates of admissions to inpatient units were requested as a combination of admissions to community-based psychiatric inpatient units in general hospitals and mental hospitals.

Rates per 100 000 population vary from 1301 in Romania and 1240 in Germany to 87 in Albania (Table 6.3, Fig. 6.3). The median rate of admissions is 568 per 100 000 population.

Table 6.2. Median number of days spent in mental hospitals and in community psychiatric inpatient units in countries

	Length of stay (days)	
Country	Mental hospitals	Community-based psychiatric inpatient units
Albania	172	19
Austria	19	11
Belgium	36	14
Bosnia and Herzegovina		
Federation of Bosnia and Herzegovina	21 (acute mental hospital in Sarajevo)	Information not available
Republika Srpska	21	11
Bulgaria	36	Information not available
Cyprus	102	11
Czech Republic	79	21
Denmark	Information not available	30
Finland	38	Information not available
Georgia	82	Not applicable
Germany	Included in community-based units	37
Greece	40	15
Ireland	18	13
Italy	Not applicable	14
Latvia	61	44
Moldova	34	Not applicable
Poland	23	Information not available
Russian Federation	77	77
Serbia	31–153 (longest in large psychiatric hospitals)	Information not available
Slovakia	Information not available	20
Slovenia	43	Information not available
Spain		
Castilla y Léon	Information not available	15
Catalonia	49	Information not available
Sweden	Information not available	25
The former Yugoslav Republic of Macedonia	260	20
Uzbekistan	42	14

Table 6.3. Admissions to inpatient units per 100 000 population in community-based psychiatric inpatient units in general hospitals and mental hospitals in countries

Country	Admissions
Albania	87
Austria	700
Azerbaijan	110
Belgium	900
Bosnia and Herzegovina	
Federation of Bosnia and Herzegovina	359
Republika Srpska	336
Bulgaria	538
Croatia	978
Cyprus	Information not available
Czech Republic	593
Denmark	730
Estonia	1150
Finland	900
France	1020
Georgia	Information not available
Germany	1240
Greece	355
Hungary	1151
Ireland	543
Israel	306
Italy	758
Latvia	835
Lithuania	674
Luxembourg	Information not available
Malta	291
Moldova	635
Montenegro	98
Netherlands	523
Norway	Information not available
Poland	646
Portugal	194
Romania	1301
Russian Federation	464
Serbia	Information not available
Slovakia	690
Slovenia	541
Spain	
Castilla y Léon	184
Catalonia	320
Extremadura	261
Galicia	151
Murcia	207
Sweden	1200
Switzerland	Information not available
The former Yugoslav Republic of Macedonia	208
Turkey	115
United Kingdom	
England and Wales	286
Scotland	543
Uzbekistan	223

Fig. 6.3. Admissions to inpatient units (mental hospitals, community psychiatric inpatient units and units in district general hospitals) per 100 000 population in countries

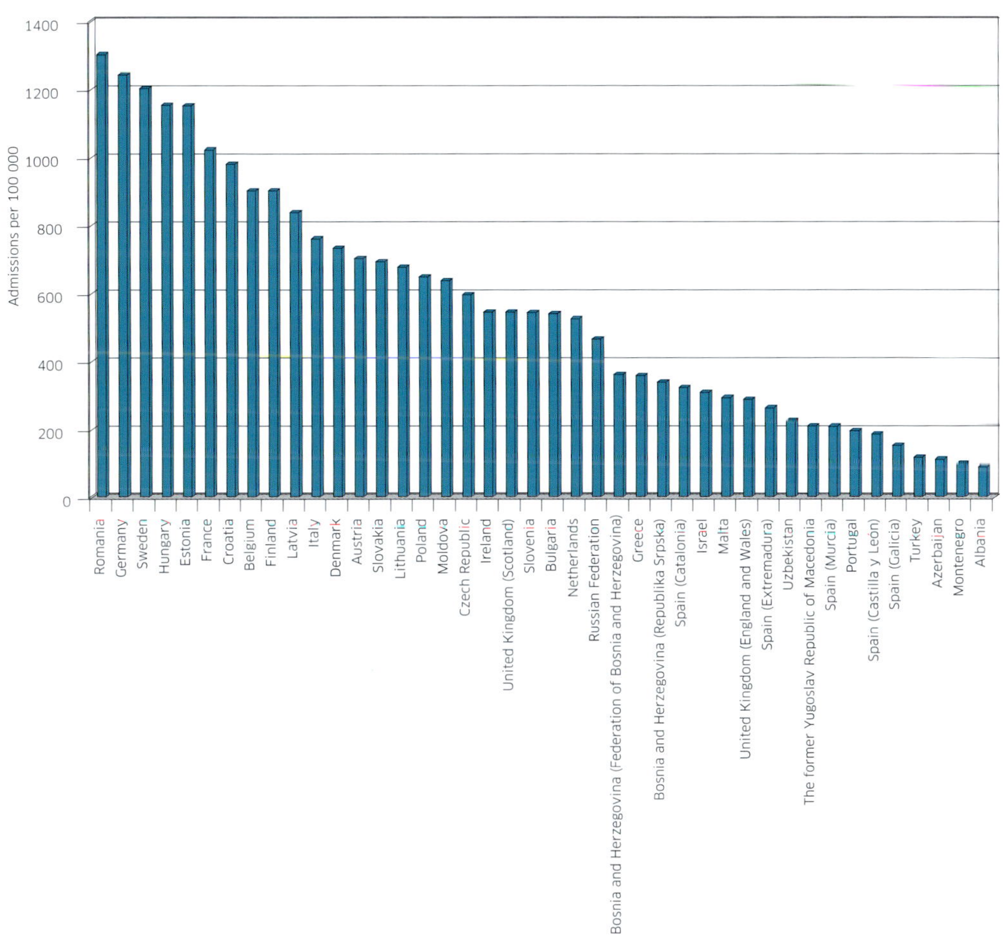

There are various reasons why countries do not have data available. Sometimes information is not reliable, and sometimes it is the wrong information.

- Finland: in 2005, 610 per 100 000 inhabitants were admitted at least once (the sex ratio was 1:1). The rate of admissions is higher (900 per 100 000), as a person may be admitted more than once.
- Georgia: the admission rate is not available. The rate of registered patients is 27.5 per 100 000 population.
- Norway: the data about admissions to inpatient units cannot be collected. The annual number of days in inpatient units is 1 689 000 for the whole population. The rate for adults receiving services from the specialized mental health units is 3% of the total population, with about 70% in outpatient units and 30% in inpatient units. For children it is 96% in outpatient care and 4% in inpatient treatment units.

Outpatient services

Availability of specialized mental health facilities

Mental health outpatient facilities

Definition

This survey defined a mental health outpatient facility as a facility that focuses on managing mental disorders and the clinical and social problems related to it on an outpatient basis.

Mental health outpatient facilities include: community mental health centres; mental health ambulatories; outpatient services for specific mental disorders or for specialized treatment; mental health outpatient departments in general hospitals; mental health polyclinics; and specialized nongovernmental organization clinics that have mental health staff and provide mental health outpatient care (such as for people who have been raped or homeless people). Both public and private not-for-profit and for-profit facilities are included. Mental health outpatient facilities for children and adolescents only and mental health outpatient facilities for other specific groups (such as older people) are also included.

Mental health outpatient facilities exclude: private practice; and facilities that solely treat people with alcohol and substance abuse disorder or mental retardation without an accompanying diagnosis of mental disorder.

This definition is broad, and it is therefore not surprising that all countries have mental health outpatient facilities available. Such facilities can differ considerably. In the CIS countries and the countries in south-eastern Europe, outpatient services are provided in polyclinics or dispensaries. Psychiatrists typically operate in small offices within larger general clinics that often also include primary care and a range of specialist services. Few support personnel are available, and treatment relies on medication.

Examples include the following.

- Bulgaria: there are 12 regional community mental health centres (dispensaries) that were established more than 30 years ago. There are also private mental health outpatient practices, but information is not available.
- Romania: according to new legislation, former outpatient services are to be transformed into community-based mental health centres. The services currently provided are prescription of monthly medication and occasionally talking therapy. Typically staffed with psychiatrists and nurses (nurses mainly deal with paperwork). As reported, many times patients queue for hours; the duration of the consultation is typically short, but it depends on the psychiatrist.

In many EU countries, outpatient clinics are offered in a department of the mental hospital or district general hospital or in purpose-build units, sometimes in community settings. Depending on the stage of development of the mental health workforce, nurses, psychologists, social workers and occupational therapists support psychiatrists.

In countries with the most developed mental health services, the concept of outpatient care has become very fluid. Appointments can be made with any member of the multidisciplinary team offered in a range of settings, including the primary care clinic. A wide range of interventions is available.

The questionnaire asked about the catchment area for the outpatient facilities, defined as the geographical area from which a service can expect to receive service users and on which the designated population of the service is based. The data provided by countries is limited due to a few main reasons. In some countries services are not organized by catchment area. In other countries the catchment area or average population covered is not even.

- Bosnia and Herzegovina (Federation of Bosnia and Herzegovina): the population covered by each service varies between regions. Outpatient services tend to be in the capitals of subregions or cities.

- Georgia: 19 outpatient facilities (psychiatric and neurological dispensaries). Mental health outpatient facilities are distributed unevenly among the regions. Each outpatient clinic serves a very different number of people. For example, a psychiatric and neurological dispensary in Tbilisi (the capital) serves about 1.3 million people.
- Norway: variation is substantial: from 23 000 to 100 000 inhabitants per facility.

Day treatment facilities

Definition

This survey defined a mental health day treatment facility as a facility that typically provides care for service users during the day. The facilities are generally:

- available to groups of users at the same time (rather than delivering services to individuals one at a time),
- expect users to stay at the facilities beyond the periods during which they have face-to-face contact with staff (that is, the service is not simply based on users coming for appointments with staff and then leaving immediately after the appointment) and
- involve attendance lasting a half day or one full day.

Day treatment facilities include: day centres; day care centres; sheltered workshops; club houses; drop in centres; and employment and rehabilitation workshops. Both public and private not-for-profit and for-profit facilities are included.

Day treatment facilities exclude: facilities that solely treat people with a diagnosis of alcohol and substance abuse disorder or intellectual disability without an accompanying diagnosis of mental disorder; general facilities that are important for people with mental disorders but that are not planned with their specific needs in mind; and day treatment facilities for inpatients.

All countries report having day treatment facilities except Cyprus, Malta, Moldova and Montenegro. Day treatment facilities mean different things in different countries.

- Bosnia and Herzegovina (Federation of Bosnia and Herzegovina): they are attached to the long-term and acute mental hospitals. Most services are focused on psychosocial rehabilitation and group therapy.
- France: there are day hospitals (65 259 places), part-time therapeutic welcome centres (92 997 places) and therapeutic workshops (5771 places).
- Serbia: day treatment facilities exist in all major cities in Serbia as part of psychiatric services.

In some countries, day treatment facilities are just being established.

- Georgia: there is only one day treatment facility in the country.
- Romania: there are only a few day treatment facilities, typically established as part of pilot initiatives in partnership with nongovernmental organizations but linked to public specialist services and then taken over by the public services, such as the Trepte Centre linked to Prof. Dr. Alexandru Obregia Clinical Psychiatric Hospital or the Titan Centre within the “Dr. Constantin Gorgos” Psychiatric Hospital in Bucharest, which was established as part of the South-eastern Europe Mental Health Project coordinated by WHO.

Visits to mental health outpatient facilities

Countries were asked to provide information on the rate of visits to all outpatient facilities per 100 000 population (Table 6.4, Fig. 6.4). In countries for which information was available, the rate varies from 28 200 in Slovakia and 26 077 in Finland to 1083 in Albania and 1066 in the United Kingdom (Scotland). The median rate is 6596.

- Bulgaria: the number of outpatient visits is not known because many service users visit private clinics that have no contract with the National Health Insurance Fund that are not reported for any statistical purposes. Some of the outpatient settings – the community mental health centres (dispensaries) – have no contract with National Health Insurance Fund and do not report this information. The settings that have a contract with National Health Insurance Fund do not provide reliable information (number of visits per month or year).
- Finland: the rate in Table 6.4. refers to visits in specialized mental health services only. It does not include visits to mental health professionals (such as psychologists and psychiatric nurses) in primary care. The rate of such visits in 2005 was 13 182 per 100 000 population. Taken together, the rate would be 39 259 visits per 100 000. The sex ratio is not available.
- Russian Federation: additional visits are not for mental disorders but to get a certificate for driving licence or a licence for weapons or family members for consultations, etc.

Fig. 6.4. Visits to outpatient facilities per 100 000 population in countries

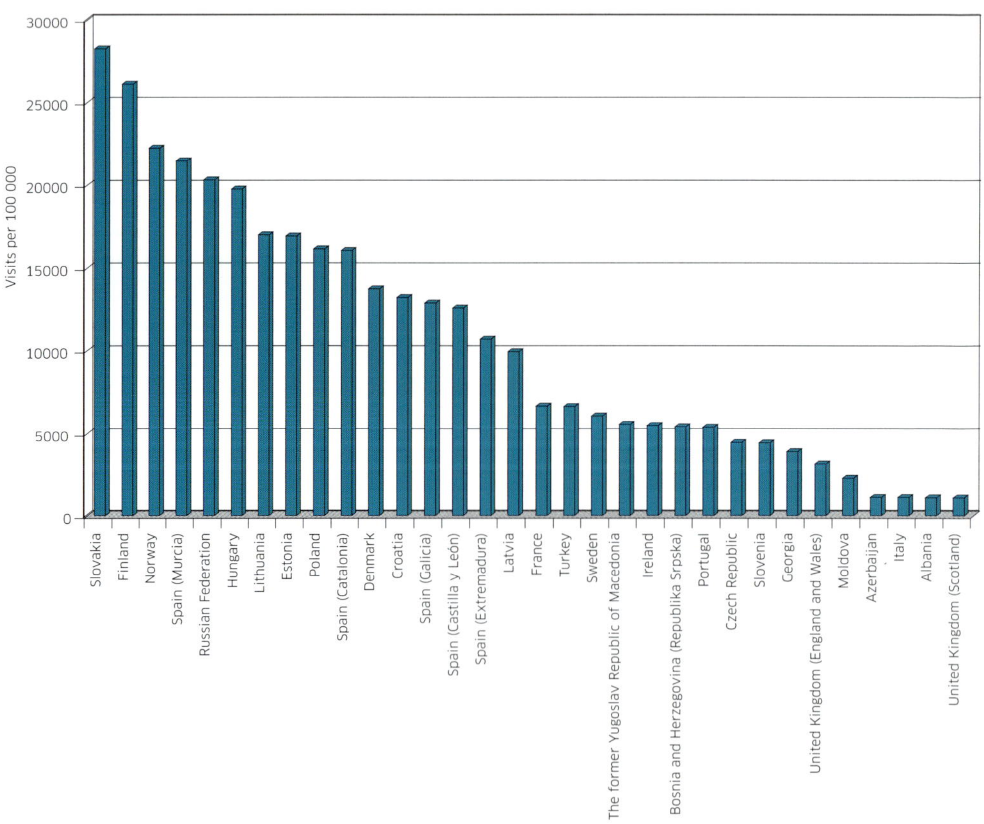

Table 6.4. Visits to mental health outpatient facilities per 100 000 population in countries

Country	Visits
Albania	1 083
Austria	Information not available
Azerbaijan	1 091
Belgium	Information not available
Bosnia and Herzegovina	
Federation of Bosnia and Herzegovina	Information not available
Republika Srpska	5 351
Bulgaria	Information not available
Croatia	13 181
Cyprus	Information not available
Czech Republic	4 399
Denmark	13 700
Estonia	16 888
Finland	26 077
France	6 612
Georgia	3 854
Germany	Information not available
Greece	Information not available
Hungary	19 726
Ireland	5 429
Israel	Information not available
Italy	1 090
Latvia	9 890
Lithuania	16 980
Luxembourg	Information not available
Malta	Information not available
Moldova	2 253
Montenegro	Information not available
Netherlands	Information not available
Norway	22 200
Poland	16 117
Portugal	5 323
Romania	Information not available
Russian Federation	20 281
Serbia	Information not available
Slovakia	28 200
Slovenia	4 387
Spain	
Castilla y Léon	12 529
Catalonia	16 009
Extremadura	10 655
Galicia	12 842
Murcia	21 428
Sweden	6 000
Switzerland	Information not available
The former Yugoslav Republic of Macedonia	5 500
Turkey	6 596
United Kingdom	
England and Wales	3 103
Scotland	1 066
Uzbekistan	Information not available

Community-based specialist mental health treatment and care

Definition
This study defined community mental health services as secondary or specialist care (care that cannot be provided by a primary care physician). At its most basic, it may be office-based private care or, more often, outpatient clinic (polyclinic) provision for assessing and treating mental illness by a trained mental health professional (such as a psychiatrist or psychologist). It can also be provided by a multidisciplinary team (community mental health team) comprising psychiatrists, mental health nurses and often psychologists and social workers. They usually provide care for the inhabitants of a clearly defined catchment area (such as a borough or town). Care is provided in a variety of settings (such as clinics, people's homes and day centres). An alternative structure is the community mental health centre, where several teams run a range of services, one of which is assessment and care outside the hospital.

Different types of community services can be distinguished. In many of the countries joining the EU since 2004, countries in south-eastern Europe and CIS countries, community services are typically provided in polyclinics or dispensaries with a psychiatric office. Nongovernmental organizations or international organizations are implementing a very small number of pilot community centres or crisis teams in some of these countries. For example, Latvia reported that people with mental disorders have full access to health care facilities in the community. Special services in the community include some day centres, ambulatories inside mental hospitals, outpatient psychiatric consultation in local community health care centres or cabinets, rehabilitation in community day centres and mental hospitals and a psychiatric centre inside a primary health care centre (one in Riga, Latvia).

Some EU15 countries have complex community-based services provided by a number of multidisciplinary teams offering crisis care, home treatment, assertive outreach and rehabilitation. Well-known examples are England and Italy, but such services are also available in countries such as Denmark, the Netherlands and Norway. Ireland says that *A vision for change* notes that the development of functioning community mental health teams is necessary to allow the provision of community-based programmes in all specialties, including home-based and assertive outreach care, as alternatives to inpatient care.

Countries were asked to indicate whether policies, plans or legislation require that people with mental disorders have access to a set of specialist mental health services in the community and the proportion of people with mental disorders who have access in practice to these services. The information provided is often indicative, since information on the use of services by people with mental health problems is limited in most countries.

- Italy: data are gathered based on studies. Only a few regions have a fully working information system.
- Spain (Castilla y León): these are routine services in clinical practice, but there is no information available on the volume of these activities.
- Sweden: about 10% of the population have a mental disorder, and about 3–4% seek psychiatric treatment each year.
- Switzerland: these are estimates based on practical experience. Statistical information is not available in Switzerland. Epidemiological data on actual need is lacking; whether this need could be met by the relevant institutions is questionable.
- United Kingdom (Scotland): breakdown is not readily available centrally, but the services described reflect the spectrum of provision and attention to mental health services in Scotland.

Community-based crisis care – daytime only

Definition
In this survey, crisis care refers to interventions that deal with brief, acute breakdowns in which an individual's usual coping strategies are temporarily overwhelmed. Early approaches tried to restrict crisis to disorders lasting days (typically 72 hours), but now care generally stretches up to several weeks. Crisis care is characterized by the rapid provision of support (such as counselling or respite admission) while arousal and distress settle and more long-term care is planned. Contact is often very frequent, sometimes more than once a day.

Policies, plans or legislation in 32 of 42 countries (76%) require that crisis care during daytime be available for people with mental disorders (Table 6.5). In practice, all or almost all people (81–100%) have access in 16 of 42 countries (38%). Seven countries (17%) report that no one has access to crisis care during daytime, and another five countries (12%) could not provide information on this (Table 6.6).

Examples of such services include the following.

- Bosnia and Herzegovina (Federation of Bosnia and Herzegovina): there are emergency rooms in hospitals. Some community mental health centres provide crisis interventions (usually psychiatrist and nurses). Some centres have good mobile services.
- Croatia: community-based crisis care – daytime only is provided by psychiatrists and mental health nurses in community-based facilities (general hospitals, outpatient clinics, health care centres and a pilot mental health care centre) as well as social workers in community-based facilities (social care centres).
- Serbia: crisis care is available at the Belgrade Institute of Mental Health and Institute of Psychiatry during the day and in large psychiatric hospitals (five of them in Serbia) 24 hours a day.

Table 6.5. Requirements for and access to community-based mental health care in crisis situations during daytime in groups of countries

Community-based crisis care (daytime)	EU		EU15		New EU countries since 2004		Israel, Norway and Switzerland		South-eastern Europe		CIS		Total	
	No.	%	No.	%	No.	%	No.	%	No.	%	No.	%	No.	%
Required in policies, plans or legislation														
Yes	22	81	13	87	9	75	3	100	6	86	1	20	32	76
No	5	19	2	13	3	25	0	0	0	0	4	80	9	21
Information not available	0	0	0	0	0	0	0	0	1	14	0	0	1	2
People with mental disorders who have access														
All or almost all (81–100%)	10	37	9	60	1	8	3	100	2	29	1	20	16	38
Majority (51–80%)	2	7	1	7	1	8	0	0	2	29	0	0	4	10
Some (21–50%)	3	11	2	13	1	8	0	0	2	29	1	20	6	14
A few (1–20%)	3	11	0	0	3	25	0	0	0	0	1	20	4	10
None	5	19	1	7	4	33	0	0	0	0	2	40	7	17
Information not available	4	15	2	13	2	17	0	0	1	14	0	0	5	12

Table 6.6. Access to community-based crisis care in daytime in countries

Country	Crisis care in daytime required in policies, plans or legislation	Percentage of people with mental disorders who have access in practice to crisis care in daytime
Albania	Yes	Some (21-50%)
Austria	No	Some (21-50%)
Azerbaijan	No	None
Belgium	Yes	All or almost all (81-100%)
Bosnia and Herzegovina		
Federation of Bosnia and Herzegovina	Yes	The majority (51-80%)
Republika Srpska	Yes	The majority (51-80%)
Bulgaria	Yes	A few (1-20%)
Croatia	Yes	All or almost all (81-100%)
Cyprus	Yes	None
Czech Republic	No	A few (1-20%)
Denmark	Yes	All or almost all (81-100%)
Estonia	Yes	All or almost all (81-100%)
Finland	Yes	Some (21-50%)
France	Yes	All or almost all (81-100%)
Georgia	No	None
Germany	Yes	All or almost all (81-100%)
Greece	Yes	None
Hungary	No	Information not available
Ireland	Yes	The majority (51-80%)
Israel	Yes	All or almost all (81-100%)
Italy	Yes	All or almost all (81-100%)
Latvia	Yes	None
Lithuania	Yes	None
Luxembourg	Yes	All or almost all (81-100%)
Malta	Yes	None
Moldova	No	Some (21-50%)
Montenegro	Yes	Some (21-50%)
Netherlands	Yes	All or almost all (81-100%)
Norway	Yes	All or almost all (81-100%)
Poland	Yes	Information not available
Portugal	No	Information not available
Romania	Yes	A few (1-20%)
Russian Federation	No	All or almost all (81-100%)
Serbia	Yes	All or almost all (81-100%)
Slovakia	Yes	The majority (51-80%)
Slovenia	No	Some (21-50%)
Spain		
Castilla y León	Yes	All or almost all (81-100%)
Catalonia	Yes	All or almost all (81-100%)
Extremadura	Yes	All or almost all (81-100%)
Galicia	Yes	All or almost all (81-100%)
Murcia	Yes	All or almost all (81-100%)
Sweden	Yes	Information not available
Switzerland	Yes	All or almost all (81-100%)
The former Yugoslav Republic of Macedonia	Yes	The majority (51-80%)
Turkey	Information not available	Information not available
United Kingdom		
England and Wales	Yes	All or almost all (81-100%)
Scotland	Yes	Information not available
Uzbekistan	Yes	A few (1-20%)

Table 6.7. Requirements for and access to community-based mental health care in crisis situations 24 hours a day in groups of countries

Community-based crisis care (24 hours a day)	EU		EU15		New EU countries since 2004		Israel, Norway and Switzerland		South-eastern Europe		CIS		Total	
	No.	%	No.	%	No.	%	No.	%	No.	%	No.	%	No.	%
Required in policies, plans or legislation														
Yes	22	81	13	87	9	75	3	100	7	100	3	60	35	83
No	5	19	2	13	3	25	0	0	0	0	2	40	7	17
People with mental disorders who have access														
All or almost all (81–100%)	10	37	8	53	2	17	3	100	0	0	2	40	15	36
Majority (51–80%)	0	0	0	0	0	0	0	0	1	14	0	0	1	2
Some (21–50%)	4	15	2	13	2	17	0	0	3	43	1	20	8	19
A few (1–20%)	4	15	1	7	3	25	0	0	0	0	0	0	4	10
None	4	15	1	7	3	25	0	0	1	14	2	40	7	17
Information not available	5	19	3	20	2	17	0	0	2	29	0	0	7	17

Community-based crisis care – 24 hours

Policies or legislation in 35 of 42 countries (83%) theoretically guarantee access to crisis care 24 hours a day (Table 6.7). Only 15 of 42 countries (36%) report that everyone with mental disorders has access to 24-hour crisis services in practice (Table 6.8).

The answers might be misleading due to different standards of what is considered crisis care in the community. All countries are likely to have emergency rooms in mental hospitals or general hospitals, but 7 of 42 countries reported the absence of 24-hour crisis services. This includes four EU countries: Greece, Lithuania, Malta and Romania. In contrast, such countries as Estonia, Hungary, the Russian Federation and Uzbekistan report that 80–100% of people with mental disorders have access to these services.

- Hungary: crisis care 24 hours – Association of the Hungarian Emergency Telephone Services.
- Latvia: no specialist psychiatric crisis centre, but in Riga emergency care by ambulance or emergency psychiatrist is available. It is possible to call 112 and the psychiatrist will come and offer a consultation and prescribe medication. Home treatment is provided only partly due to lack of resources.

Table 6.8. Access to community-based crisis care 24 hours a day in countries

Country	Crisis care 24 hours a day required in policies, plans or legislation	Percentage of people with mental disorders who have access in practice to crisis care 24 hours a day
Albania	Yes	Some (21-50%)
Austria	No	Some (21-50%)
Azerbaijan	Yes	None
Belgium	Yes	All or almost all (81-100%)
Bosnia and Herzegovina		
Federation of Bosnia and Herzegovina	Yes	The majority (51-80%)
Republika Srpska	Yes	The majority (51-80%)
Bulgaria	Yes	A few (1-20%)
Croatia	Yes	Some (21-50%)
Cyprus	Yes	Information not available
Czech Republic	No	A few (1-20%)
Denmark	Yes	All or almost all (81-100%)
Estonia	Yes	All or almost all (81-100%)
Finland	No	A few (1-20%)
France	Yes	Information not available
Georgia	No	None
Germany	Yes	All or almost all (81-100%)
Greece	Yes	None
Hungary	Yes	All or almost all (81-100%)
Ireland	Yes	Some (21-50%)
Israel	Yes	All or almost all (81-100%)
Italy	Yes	All or almost all (81-100%)
Latvia	No	Some (21-50%)
Lithuania	Yes	None
Luxembourg	Yes	All or almost all (81-100%)
Malta	Yes	None
Moldova	Yes	Some (21-50%)
Montenegro	Yes	Some (21-50%)
Netherlands	Yes	All or almost all (81-100%)
Norway	Yes	All or almost all (81-100%)
Poland	Yes	Information not available
Portugal	Yes	Information not available
Romania	No	None
Russian Federation	Yes	All or almost all (81-100%)
Serbia	Yes	Information not available
Slovakia	Yes	Some (21-50%)
Slovenia	Yes	A few (1-20%)
Spain		
Castilla y León	Yes	All or almost all (81-100%)
Catalonia	Yes	A few (1-20%)
Extremadura	Yes	All or almost all (81-100%)
Galicia	Yes	All or almost all (81-100%)
Murcia	Yes	All or almost all (81-100%)
Sweden	Yes	Information not available
Switzerland	Yes	All or almost all (81-100%)
The former Yugoslav Republic of Macedonia	Yes	None
Turkey	Yes	Information not available
United Kingdom		
England and Wales	Yes	All or almost all (81-100%)
Scotland	Yes	Information not available
Uzbekistan	No	All or almost all (81-100%)

Home treatment

Definition
Few mental health interventions require complex equipment or specialized accommodation. Treatment (psychological, pharmaceutical and social) is increasingly provided in the person's home or neighbourhood when it is safe to do so. Home treatment often implies that the intervention has an acknowledged aim of diverting the person away from hospital admission and may involve frequent contact (usually between daily and weekly).

Of the 42 countries, 33 (79%) report that access to home treatment for people with mental disorders is expected in policies, plans or legislation (Table 6.9). In practice, only Germany, Luxembourg and the United Kingdom (England and Wales) report that all or almost all people with mental disorders have access to home treatment. In eight countries this service is not available, and another eight countries could not provide information on the proportion of people actually having access to home treatment (Table 6.10).

- Poland: community mobile teams (29 in 2005) provide home treatment.
- Russian Federation: home treatment can be difficult in remote areas.
- Serbia: home treatment is organized at the Institute of Mental Health (and has been since it was established 45 years ago) with mobile teams consisting of a psychiatrist, nurse and social worker.

Table 6.9. Requirements for and access to mental health home treatment in groups of countries

Home treatment	EU		EU15		New EU countries since 2004		Israel, Norway and Switzerland		South-eastern Europe		CIS		Total	
	No.	%	No.	%	No.	%	No.	%	No.	%	No.	%	No.	%
Required in policies, plans or legislation														
Yes	21	78	14	93	7	58	3	100	6	86	3	60	33	79
No	6	22	1	7	5	42	0	0	0	0	2	40	8	19
Information not available	0	0	0	0	0	0	0	0	1	14	0	0	1	2
People with mental disorders who have access														
All or almost all (81–100%)	3	11	3	20	0	0	0	0	0	0	0	0	3	7
Majority (51–80%)	1	4	1	7	0	0	1	33	0	0	1	20	3	7
Some (21–50%)	5	19	4	27	1	8	2	67	3	43	1	20	11	26
A few (1–20%)	6	22	3	20	3	25	0	0	2	29	1	20	9	21
None	5	19	0	0	5	42	0	0	1	14	2	40	8	19
Information not available	7	26	4	27	3	25	0	0	1	14	0	0	8	19

Table 6.10. Access to home treatment in countries

Country	Home treatment required in policies, plans or legislation	Percentage of people with mental disorders who have access in practice to home treatment
Albania	Yes	Some (21–50%)
Austria	No	Information not available
Azerbaijan	No	None
Belgium	Yes	Some (21–50%)
Bosnia and Herzegovina		
Federation of Bosnia and Herzegovina	Yes	Some (21–50%)
Republika Srpska	Yes	Some (21–50%)
Bulgaria	Yes	None
Croatia	Yes	None
Cyprus	Yes	Information not available
Czech Republic	Yes	None
Denmark	Yes	Some (21–50%)
Estonia	No	A few (1–20%)
Finland	Yes	A few (1–20%)
France	Yes	Information not available
Georgia	No	None
Germany	Yes	All or almost all (81–100%)
Greece	Yes	A few (1–20%)
Hungary	No	None
Ireland	Yes	Some (21–50%)
Israel	Yes	The majority (51–80%)
Italy	Yes	Some (21–50%)
Latvia	Yes	Some (21–50%)
Lithuania	Yes	A few (1–20%)
Luxembourg	Yes	All or almost all (81–100%)
Malta	Yes	None
Moldova	Yes	Some (21–50%)
Montenegro	Yes	A few (1–20%)
Netherlands	Yes	The majority (51–80%)
Norway	Yes	Some (21–50%)
Poland	Yes	A few (1–20%)
Portugal	Yes	Information not available
Romania	No	None
Russian Federation	Yes	The majority (51–80%)
Serbia	Yes	A few (1–20%)
Slovakia	No	Information not available
Slovenia	No	Information not available
Spain		
Castilla y León	Yes	Information not available
Catalonia	Yes	A few (1–20%)
Extremadura	Yes	A few (1–20%)
Galicia	Yes	A few (1–20%)
Murcia	No	A few (1–20%)
Sweden	Yes	Information not available
Switzerland	Yes	Some (21–50%)
The former Yugoslav Republic of Macedonia	Yes	Some (21–50%)
Turkey	Information not available	Information not available
United Kingdom		
England and Wales	Yes	All or almost all (81–100%)
Scotland	Yes	Information not available
Uzbekistan	Yes	A few (1–20%)

Assertive outreach

> **Definition**
> Assertive outreach has been defined as community-based services that work intensively over time with people with complex mental health needs addressing mental health, physical health and social needs.

Of the 42 countries, 22 (52%) have policy, plans or legislation requiring that people with mental disorders have access to assertive outreach services (Table 6.11). Only the United Kingdom (England and Wales) reports that all people with mental disorders have access to these services, and 16 of 42 countries (38%) report that they do not provide assertive outreach services (Table 6.12). The scale of provision between England and Wales and the other countries differs considerably.

- In Albania, assertive outreach is one of the tasks of the new community mental health centres, but it covers only a small proportion of the population.
- Norway: there is an effort to offer increasing access to assertive outreach teams and early intervention, and the outpatient and inpatient units are expected to have this resource available.

Table 6.11. Requirements for and access to assertive outreach for people with complex mental health needs in groups of countries

Assertive outreach	EU		EU15		New EU countries since 2004		Israel, Norway and Switzerland		South-eastern Europe		CIS		Total	
	No.	%	No.	%	No.	%	No.	%	No.	%	No.	%	No.	%
Required in policies, plans or legislation														
Yes	15	56	12	80	3	25	2	67	3	43	2	40	22	52
No	10	37	3	20	7	58	1	33	3	43	3	60	17	40
Information not available	2	7	0	0	2	17	0	0	1	14	0	0	3	7
People with complex needs who have access														
All or almost all (81-100%)	1	4	1	7	0	0	0	0	0	0	0	0	1	2
Majority (51-80%)	2	7	2	13	0	0	0	0	0	0	1	20	3	7
Some (21-50%)	3	11	3	20	0	0	1	33	0	0	0	0	4	10
A few (1-20%)	5	19	3	20	2	17	2	67	3	43	1	20	11	26
None	10	37	2	13	8	67	0	0	3	43	3	60	16	38
Information not available	6	22	4	27	2	17	0	0	1	14	0	0	7	17

Table 6.12. Access to assertive outreach in countries

Country	Assertive outreach required in policies, plans or legislation	Percentage of people with mental disorders who have access in practice to assertive outreach
Albania	Yes	A few (1-20%)
Austria	No	None
Azerbaijan	No	None
Belgium	Yes	Some (21-50%)
Bosnia and Herzegovina		
Federation of Bosnia and Herzegovina	No	None
Republika Srpska	No	Information not available
Bulgaria	Yes	None
Croatia	No	None
Cyprus	No	None
Czech Republic	No	None
Denmark	Yes	The majority (51-80%)
Estonia	No	A few (1-20%)
Finland	No	A few (1-20%)
France	Yes	Information not available
Georgia	No	None
Germany	Yes	The majority (51-80%)
Greece	No	None
Hungary	No	None
Ireland	Yes	Some (21-50%)
Israel	No	A few (1-20%)
Italy	Yes	A few (1-20%)
Latvia	No	None
Lithuania	Information not available	None
Luxembourg	Yes	Information not available
Malta	Yes	A few (1-20%)
Moldova	Yes	A few (1-20%)
Montenegro	No	None
Netherlands	Yes	Some (21-50%)
Norway	Yes	Some (21-50%)
Poland	Yes	Information not available
Portugal	Yes	Information not available
Romania	No	None
Russian Federation	Yes	The majority (51-80%)
Serbia	Yes	A few (1-20%)
Slovakia	No	None
Slovenia	Information not available	Information not available
Spain		
Castilla y León	Yes	The majority (51-80%)
Catalonia	Yes	A few (1-20%)
Extremadura	Yes	None
Galicia	Yes	None
Murcia	Yes	A few (1-20%)
Sweden	Yes	Information not available
Switzerland	Yes	A few (1-20%)
The former Yugoslav Republic of Macedonia	Yes	A few (1-20%)
Turkey	Information not available	Information not available
United Kingdom		
England and Wales	Yes	All or almost all (81-100%)
Scotland	Yes	Information not available
Uzbekistan	No	None

Community-based early intervention

Definition

In this study, early intervention refers to providing services early in the evolution of psychoses, thereby reducing the duration of untreated psychosis. Reducing this duration is thought to contribute to better outcome. Such services are usually multidisciplinary teams that use a range of techniques, including outreach to schools and raising awareness of early signs of deterioration (prodromes). They provide intensive treatment aimed at preventing deterioration.

Policies, plans or legislation in 26 countries (62%) require that people with mental disorders have access to early interventions, but in practice only three countries (Germany, Luxembourg and the United Kingdom (England and Wales)) report that 80–100% of these people receive such services (Tables 6.13 and 6.14).

Similar to other specialist community services, the scale of implementation differs greatly. England is the only country providing a network of specialist early intervention teams countrywide targeting young people with early stages of psychotic disorders.

Switzerland offered an interesting angle, indicating the fine line between early and tertiary intervention.

The countries made the following comments.

- Switzerland: disability insurance has the aim of vocational rehabilitation ("integration before benefit"). Early inclusion and early intervention also need to consider which groups of mentally ill people should receive timely assistance to prevent their condition from becoming chronic.
- Bosnia and Herzegovina (Federation of Bosnia and Herzegovina): some early interventions from general practitioners.

Table 6.13. Requirements for and access to community-based early intervention in psychosis in groups of countries

Community-based early intervention	EU		EU15		New EU countries since 2004		Israel, Norway and Switzerland		South-eastern Europe		CIS		Total	
	No.	%	No.	%	No.	%	No.	%	No.	%	No.	%	No.	%
Required in policies, plans or legislation														
Yes	17	63	12	80	5	42	2	67	5	71	2	40	26	62
No	9	33	3	20	6	50	1	33	1	14	3	60	14	33
Information not available	1	4	0	0	1	8	0	0	1	14	0	0	2	5
People with mental disorders who have access														
All or almost all (81–100%)	3	11	3	20	0	0	0	0	0	0	0	0	3	7
Majority (51–80%)	3	11	3	20	0	0	1	33	0	0	1	20	5	12
Some (21–50%)	2	7	2	13	0	0	1	33	2	29	0	0	5	12
A few (1–20%)	5	19	2	13	3	25	0	0	2	29	2	40	9	21
None	7	26	1	7	6	50	1	33	1	14	2	40	11	26
Information not available	7	26	4	27	3	25	0	0	2	29	0	0	9	21

Table 6.14. Access to community-based early intervention in countries

Country	Early intervention required in policies, plans or legislation	Percentage of people with mental disorders who have access in practice to early intervention
Albania	Yes	A few (1–20%)
Austria	No	Information not available
Azerbaijan	No	None
Belgium	Yes	Some (21–50%)
Bosnia and Herzegovina		
Federation of Bosnia and Herzegovina	Yes	A few (1–20%)
Republika Srpska	Yes	Some (21–50%)
Bulgaria	Yes	A few (1–20%)
Croatia	No	Information not available
Cyprus	No	Information not available
Czech Republic	No	None
Denmark	Yes	The majority (51–80%)
Estonia	No	A few (1–20%)
Finland	No	A few (1–20%)
France	Yes	Information not available
Georgia	No	None
Germany	Yes	All or almost all (81–100%)
Greece	No	None
Hungary	No	None
Ireland	Yes	A few (1–20%)
Israel	No	None
Italy	Yes	The majority (51–80%)
Latvia	No	None
Lithuania	Yes	None
Luxembourg	Yes	All or almost all (81–100%)
Malta	Yes	None
Moldova	No	A few (1–20%)
Montenegro	Yes	None
Netherlands	Yes	Some (21–50%)
Norway	Yes	Some (21–50%)
Poland	Yes	Information not available
Portugal	Yes	Information not available
Romania	Yes	A few (1–20%)
Russian Federation	Yes	The majority (51–80%)
Serbia	Yes	A few (1–20%)
Slovakia	No	None
Slovenia	Information not available	Information not available
Spain		
Castilla y León	No	Information not available
Catalonia	Yes	A few (1–20%)
Extremadura	Information not available	Information not available
Galicia	Yes	The majority (51–80%)
Murcia	No	Information not available
Sweden	Yes	Information not available
Switzerland	Yes	The majority (51–80%)
The former Yugoslav Republic of Macedonia	Yes	Some (21–50%)
Turkey	Information not available	Information not available
United Kingdom		
England and Wales	Yes	All or almost all (81–100%)
Scotland	Yes	Information not available
Uzbekistan	Yes	A few (1–20%)

Community-based rehabilitation services

Most countries have policies, plans or legislation requiring that people with mental disorders have access to rehabilitation services (Table 6.15). Only two countries (Azerbaijan and Montenegro) reported that these services are not available in community settings, but 11 of 42 countries (26%) indicate that such services are available in practice for only 1–20% of the people with mental health problems, including 5 of the 12 countries that joined the EU since 2004 and 3 of the 5 CIS countries. Ten countries (24%) report that all or almost all people with mental disorders have access in practice to these services (Table 6.16).

- Bosnia and Herzegovina (Federation of Bosnia and Herzegovina): such services are provided by community-based mental health centres.
- Croatia: community-based rehabilitation services are provided by psychiatrists and mental health nurses in community-based facilities (general hospitals, outpatient clinics, health care centres and a pilot mental health care centre); in some high-resource areas, teams include occupational therapists and social workers.

Table 6.15. Requirements for and access to community-based rehabilitation services for people with mental disorders in groups of countries

Community-based rehabilitation services	EU		EU15		New EU countries since 2004		Israel, Norway and Switzerland		South-eastern Europe		CIS		Total	
	No.	%	No.	%	No.	%	No.	%	No.	%	No.	%	No.	%
Required in policies, plans or legislation														
Yes	24	89	14	93	10	83	3	100	6	86	5	100	38	90
No	1	4	1	7	0	0	0	0	0	0	0	0	1	2
Information not available	2	7	0	0	2	17	0	0	1	14	0	0	3	7
People with mental disorders who have access														
All or almost all (81–100%)	10	37	9	60	1	8	0	0	0	0	0	0	10	24
Majority (51–80%)	4	15	3	20	1	8	1	33	0	0	1	20	6	14
Some (21–50%)	1	4	0	0	1	8	2	67	3	43	0	0	6	14
A few (1–20%)	6	22	1	7	5	42	0	0	2	29	3	60	11	26
None	0	0	0	0	0	0	0	0	1	14	1	20	2	5
Information not available	6	22	2	13	4	33	0	0	1	14	0	0	7	17

Table 6.16. Access to community-based rehabilitation services in countries

Country	Rehabilitation services required in policies, plans or legislation	Percentage of people with mental disorders who have access in practice to rehabilitation services
Albania	Yes	A few (1-20%)
Austria	No	All or almost all (81-100%)
Azerbaijan	Yes	None
Belgium	Yes	All or almost all (81-100%)
Bosnia and Herzegovina		
Federation of Bosnia and Herzegovina	Yes	Some (21-50%)
Republika Srpska	Yes	Some (21-50%)
Bulgaria	Yes	A few (1-20%)
Croatia	Yes	Some (21-50%)
Cyprus	Yes	Information not available
Czech Republic	Yes	A few (1-20%)
Denmark	Yes	The majority (51-80%)
Estonia	Yes	All or almost all (81-100%)
Finland	Yes	A few (1-20%)
France	Yes	All or almost all (81-100%)
Georgia	Yes	A few (1-20%)
Germany	Yes	All or almost all (81-100%)
Greece	Yes	The majority (51-80%)
Hungary	Yes	A few (1-20%)
Ireland	Yes	The majority (51-80%)
Israel	Yes	Some (21-50%)
Italy	Yes	All or almost all (81-100%)
Latvia	Yes	A few (1-20%)
Lithuania	Yes	Information not available
Luxembourg	Yes	All or almost all (81-100%)
Malta	Yes	Some (21-50%)
Moldova	Yes	A few (1-20%)
Montenegro	Yes	None
Netherlands	Yes	All or almost all (81-100%)
Norway	Yes	The majority (51-80%)
Poland	Yes	The majority (51-80%)
Portugal	Yes	Information not available
Romania	Yes	A few (1-20%)
Russian Federation	Yes	The majority (51-80%)
Serbia	Yes	A few (1-20%)
Slovakia	Information not available	Information not available
Slovenia	Information not available	Information not available
Spain		
Castilla y León	Yes	Some (21-50%)
Catalonia	Yes	Some (21-50%)
Extremadura	Yes	All or almost all (81-100%)
Galicia	Yes	The majority (51-80%)
Murcia	Yes	All or almost all (81-100%)
Sweden	Yes	Information not available
Switzerland	Yes	Some (21-50%)
The former Yugoslav Republic of Macedonia	Yes	Some (21-50%)
Turkey	Information not available	Information not available
United Kingdom		
England and Wales	Yes	All or almost all (81-100%)
Scotland	Yes	Information not available
Uzbekistan	Yes	A few (1-20%)

Residential health facilities

Availability of specialized mental health facilities

Community residential health facilities

Definition

A community residential health facility has been defined as a non-hospital, community-based mental health facility that provides overnight residence for people with mental disorders. Usually these facilities serve users with relatively stable mental disorders not requiring intensive pharmaceutical interventions.

Community residential health facilities include: supervised housing; unstaffed group homes; group homes with some residential or visiting staff; hostels with day staff; hostels with day and night staff; hostels and homes with 24-hour nursing staff; halfway houses; and therapeutic communities. Both public and private not-for-profit and for-profit facilities are included. Community residential facilities for children and adolescents only and community residential facilities for other specific groups (such as older people) are also included.

Community residential health facilities exclude: facilities that treat only people with a diagnosis of alcohol and substance abuse disorder or mental retardation; residential facilities in mental hospitals; generic facilities that are important for people with mental disorders but that are not planned with their specific needs in mind, such as nursing homes and rest homes for older people, institutions treating mainly diseases of the nervous system or physical disability problems.

Many countries report that they do not have community residential health facilities, including Azerbaijan, Croatia, Hungary, Latvia, Lithuania, Moldova, Montenegro, Slovakia, Slovenia, the former Yugoslav Republic of Macedonia and Turkey.

Residential facilities that are not health care (social institutions)

Definition

This survey defined a residential facility that is not health care as a residential facility that houses people with mental disorders but does not meet the definition for a community residential facility or any other mental health facility defined here (community-based psychiatric inpatient unit, community residential facility, forensic inpatient unit or mental hospital).

Residential facilities that are not health care include: residential facilities specifically for people with mental retardation, for people with substance abuse problems or for people with dementia. Included are also residential facilities that are not formally mental health facilities but facilities in which most of the people residing have diagnosable mental disorders.

Social institutions are available in most European countries. Few countries provided data on social institutions, since they are typically under the authority of social welfare ministries, and the operation of these homes is often delegated to local authorities. In some countries such large facilities provide long-term care for people with all types of disability put together.

Beds in residential facilities

Beds per 100 000 population in community residential health facilities

The beds or places per 100 000 population in community residential health facilities in the 16 countries that provided information range from 93 in Israel and 80 in Ireland to 1.2 in Albania and 1 in Bosnia and Herzegovina (Republika Srpska) (Table 6.17 and Fig. 6.5).

In several countries, these represent small-scale initiatives.

Fig. 6.5. Beds in community residential health facilities per 100 000 population in countries

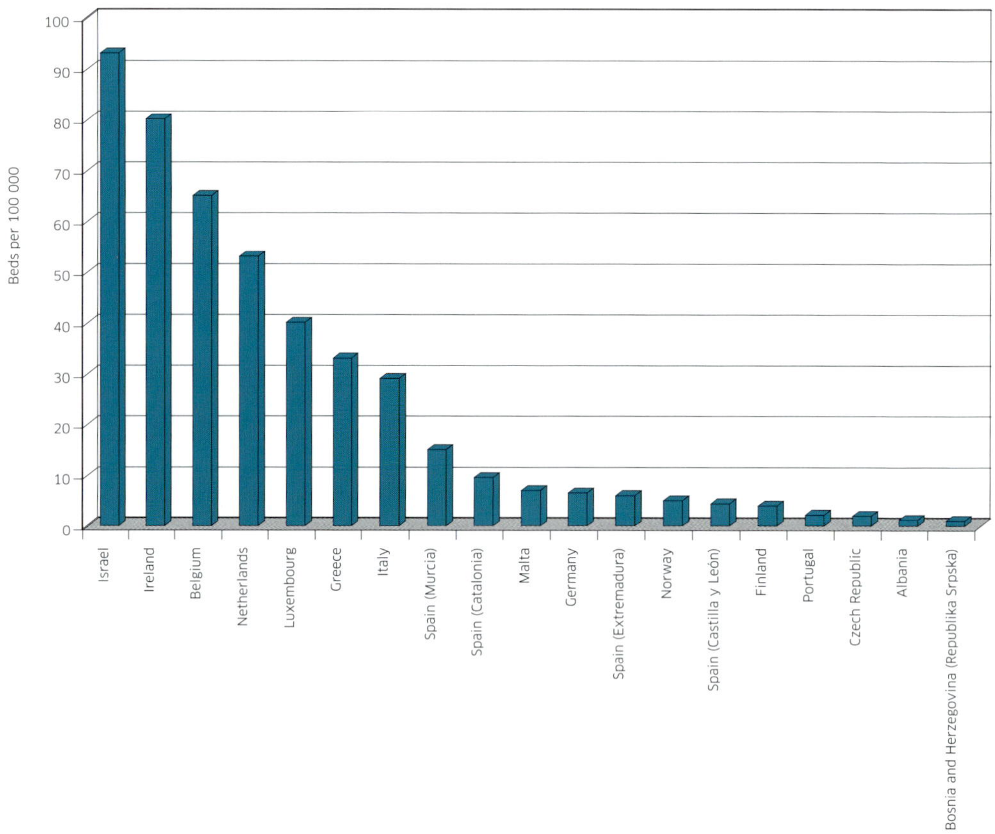

- Albania: there are 5 protected homes for 37 people with severe mental health problems. These have been pilot initiatives developed with international support from WHO and other international partners (United Nations Office for Project Services (UNOPS) and the Community of St. Egidio).
- Bosnia and Herzegovina (Federation of Bosnia and Herzegovina): there are two protected flats for eight people with mental health problems.
- Bosnia and Herzegovina (Republika Srpska): there are 2 protected flats for 14 people: safe house Kladari in Modrica for continued care clients (10 beds) and a safe flat in Doboj (4 beds).
- Bulgaria: the Ministry of Labour and Social Policy recently developed and financed some pilot initiatives.
- Czech Republic: about 200 places in supervised housing.
- Georgia: community-based alternatives to institutionalization for people with mental disability are operated as demonstration projects mainly by nongovernmental organizations. Most of these services are based in Tbilisi with very few examples functioning in other parts of the country.
- Malta: two hostels for clients previously residing in the mental hospital.
- Russian Federation: there are 10 community residential health facilities for 312 people.
- Uzbekistan: two community residential health facilities.

Table 6.17. Beds in community residential health facilities per 100 000 population in countries

Country	Beds
Albania	1.2
Belgium	65
Bosnia and Herzegovina (Republika Srpska)	1
Czech Republic	2
Finland	4
Germany	6.5
Greece	33
Ireland	80
Israel	93
Italy	29
Luxembourg	40
Malta	7
Netherlands	53
Norway	5
Portugal	2.2
Spain	
Castilla y Léon	4.4
Catalonia	9.5
Extremadura	6
Murcia	15

Table 6.18. Beds in residential facilities that are not health care (social institutions) per 100 000 population in countries

Country	Beds
Azerbaijan	12
Bosnia and Herzegovina	
Federation of Bosnia and Herzegovina	11.7
Republika Srpska	12
Bulgaria	59
Czech Republic	12
Finland	102
Georgia	3.6
Latvia	189
Netherlands	1
Poland	13
Portugal	34
Russian Federation	90
Slovakia	6
Slovenia	127
Spain	
Catalonia	3.6
Extremadura	6
Murcia	18
Sweden	80

Beds per 100 000 population in residential facilities that are not health care (social institutions)

Many countries provide residential places for persons with long term mental health problems, including social care homes, that are the responsibility of ministries other than health. Data tend to be imprecise but the table and figure below give some impression (Table 6.18 and Fig. 6.6).

- Bulgaria: for mentally disabled children around 2000 places, for youth about 1000, for adults around 4500 places for the whole country. In general, the protected homes established under the Social Assistance Agency do not provide mental health care.
- Czech Republic: social institutions for people with alcohol dependence (356 places) and social institutions for mental disorders (881 places).
- Finland: these are usually private and lack a specific catchment area.
- Georgia: there are only two social institutions - one special social ward in Zurabashvili (Gldani) psychiatric hospital with 100 beds and only one separate institution – “House for People with Intellectual and Physical Disabilities” – for 55 people in Dzevri village in western Georgia. They formally must serve the whole population of Georgia but in reality can satisfy the needs of only a small part of the population.
- Russian Federation: this figure is the number of people (all age groups) staying in psychiatric and neurological internats (residential institutions for young people).
- The former Yugoslav Republic of Macedonia: there are only residential facilities for older people.
- Uzbekistan: 13 in the system of the Ministry of Labour and Social Protection, excluding seven sanatoriums and boarding homes for older people.

Fig. 6.6. Beds in residential facilities that are not health care (social institutions) per 100 000 population in countries

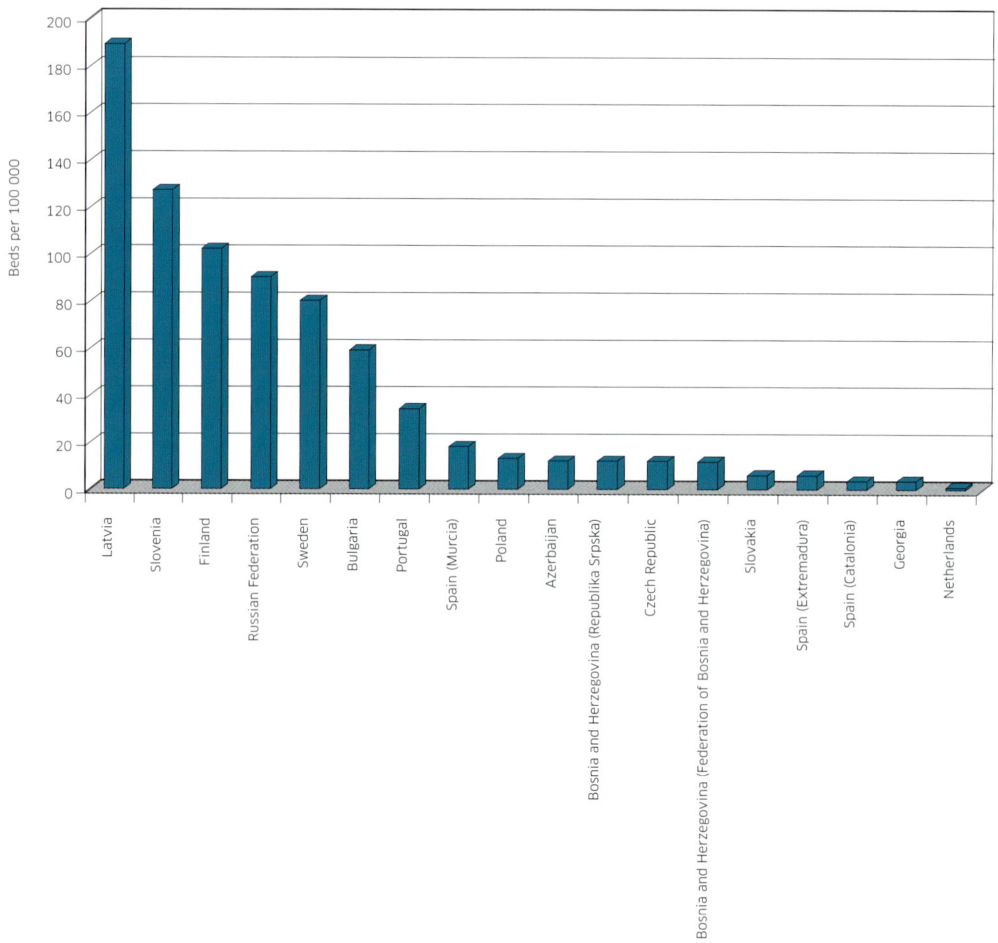

Forensic units

Definition

Forensic units care for people with mental disorders who have come into contact with the criminal justice system. They may also be called secure units or special hospitals.

The data on beds in forensic mental health units are available for 60% of the countries (Table 6.19 and Fig. 6.7). The variation is very great and could be caused by many factors. One possible explanation is that forensic hospitals serve different target groups. In some countries, such as Italy, they house clients referred by the court. In other countries such as the United Kingdom (England and Wales), residents are a combination of people referred by the courts or people transferred from other hospitals for severely challenging behaviour.

Not all countries have specified beds for forensic purposes. For example, in Denmark, the forensic units are part of the general hospitals. They are part of the general number of beds in the mental health services. There is no special legal condition about forensic units (except for one special highly secured unit); it is merely a question of practical organization.

Some people in forensic units require a higher security level and stay longer than other people. Many such people are treated in ordinary community inpatient units or in outpatient services.

- Austria: according to the Austrian penal law, the rate of 7.8 can be divided into 3.9 for "non-responsible" and 4.0 for "responsible" mentally ill offenders.
- Belgium: the number of beds in forensic units per 100 000 population is based on four pilot projects for beds in forensic units in mental hospitals that have been established during the past few years.
- Italy: the data refer to the number of people charged in 2006, which can vary according to referrals. It is not a fixed number of beds or places.

In some countries, forensic psychiatric beds are based in prisons.

- Hungary: the only forensic psychiatric unit in the country is within a prison. There are no forensic psychiatric units in general or psychiatric hospitals and there are no community forensic mental health units.
- Bosnia and Herzegovina (Federation of Bosnia and Herzegovina): there is a forensic unit in a prison with 29 beds.
- Albania: there are 35 beds placed at the prison hospital that provide treatment to people with mental disorders who have come into contact with the criminal justice system.

Table 6.19. Beds in forensic units per 100 000 population in countries

Country	Beds
Albania	1
Austria	7.8
Azerbaijan	4.3
Belgium	3
Bosnia and Herzegovina	
Federation of Bosnia and Herzegovina	1.2
Republika Srpska	7.1
Finland	8
Georgia	7.4
Germany	10.5
Greece	2.7
Ireland	1.8
Israel	2
Italy	1.8
Latvia	7
Lithuania	14
Luxembourg	0
Malta	1
Moldova	3
Netherlands	4
Poland	2
Portugal	0.2
Romania	4
Russian Federation	1.6
Slovakia	20
Spain	
Castilla y Léon	0
Catalonia	0.9
Sweden	15

Mental health services for children and adolescents

This survey enquired about the presence of specialized mental health services for children and adolescents in inpatient, outpatient and residential settings (Table 6.20). A particular challenge in this section is the very great variation in capacity and quality, which cannot be extracted from national data. Some of the examples can give some impression about the issues faced.

Inpatient facilities

Mental hospitals

Specialized services for children and adolescents are available in mental hospitals in 30 of 42 countries (71%). The examples demonstrate that such units serve different functions and sometimes have limited capacity to handle the caseloads.

- Azerbaijan: there is one division for children and adolescents in Republic Mental Health Hospital #1. These divisions work as a social institution where children stay permanently.
- Bulgaria: extremely insufficient capacity. Only two in two of the big cities – Sofia and Varna – and clinics at the large hospitals.
- Croatia: services seriously understaffed.
- Slovakia: 80 beds for all of Slovakia.
- Switzerland: there are youth psychiatric units in many cantons, as well as children's psychiatric units, which are generally linked to a special school.

Fig. 6.7. Beds in forensic units per 100 000 population in countries

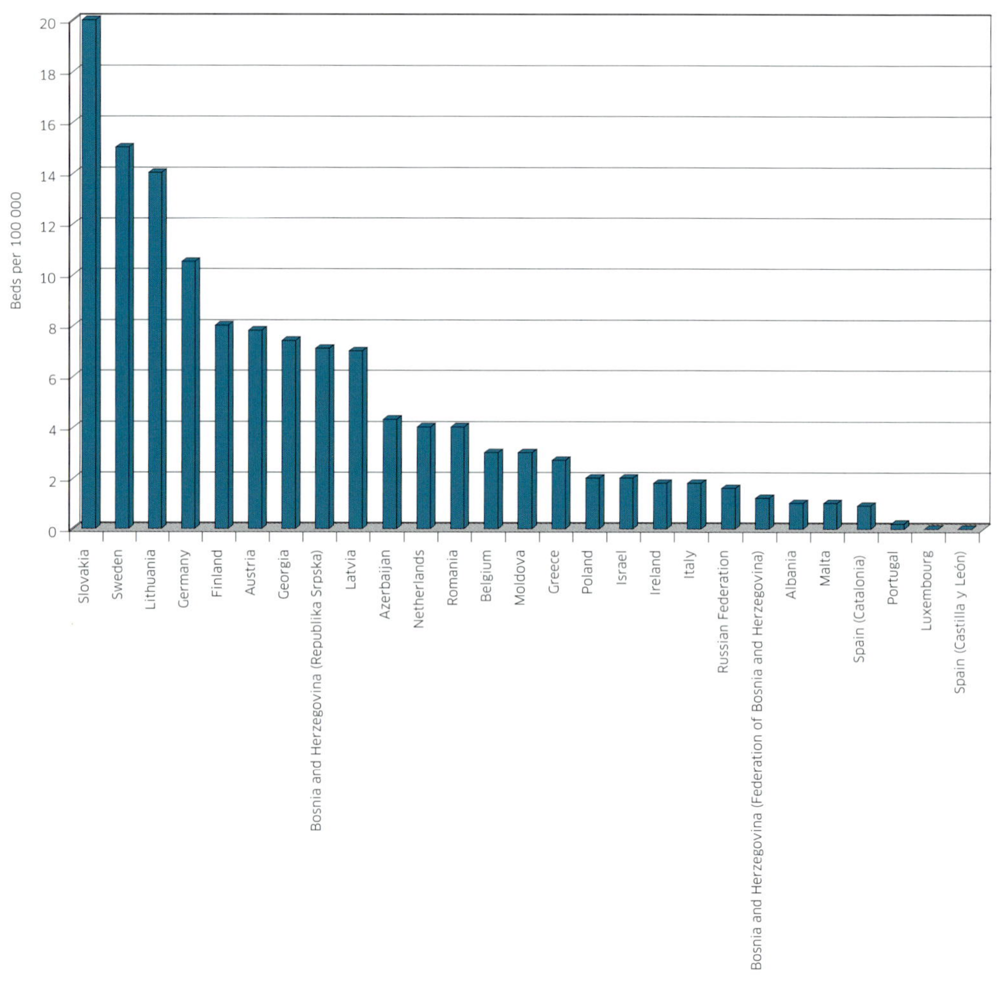

- Turkey: specialized mental health services for children and adolescents are available at Bakırköy Professor Dr Mazhar Osman Education and Research Mental Hospital (Istanbul), Dr. Ekrem Tok (Adana) Mental Hospital and Manisa Mental Hospital.

Community-based psychiatric inpatient units and units in district general hospitals
Community-based psychiatric inpatient units and units in district general hospitals provide mental health services for children and adolescents in 28 of 42 countries, including in 14 of the EU15 countries (93%) and 5 of the 12 countries that joined the EU since 2004 (42%).

- Germany: 228 child and youth psychiatric units (departments and specialized hospitals).
- Italy: there is great variation among the regions.
- Serbia: child and adolescent psychiatric units are available at the Institute of Mental Health in Belgrade (inpatient, outpatient and day hospitals). There is also a university psychiatric hospital for children in Belgrade and at all major cities with university psychiatric hospitals.
- Switzerland: not all cantons have units, but most have child psychiatric beds in paediatric units.

- Uzbekistan: child psychosomatic departments with 60 beds are functioning at Andijan, Jizzakh and Syrdarya regional child multisectoral hospitals.

Outpatient facilities

Mental health outpatient facilities

Almost all countries (40 of 42) report that specialist mental health services for children and adolescents are available in mental health outpatient facilities.

- Germany: 266 youth counselling centres.
- Ireland: mental health services for children and adolescents adopt a life-span approach and are guided by the policy A vision for change. This identifies the need for a full range of mental health services for children and adolescents across primary and specialist service provision. The objective is the provision of two multidisciplinary mental health teams for children and adolescents per 100 000 population.
- Latvia: four outpatient services for children and adolescents, each covering about 31 000 people.
- Lithuania: there are 72 mental health centres. Every centre should employ a psychiatrist specializing in children, but in some of them they are absent.
- Norway: about 4% of the children and youth in Norway are receiving specialized treatment for mental health problems, 97% of these in outpatient units.
- Slovakia: varies from region to region from 0 facilities to 2–3 facilities per 600 000 inhabitants.

Day treatment facilities

Day treatment facilities for mental health services for children and adolescents are available in 32 of 42 countries (76%), including all the EU15 countries except Sweden. Again, differences in provision are striking.

- Bulgaria: 58 centres for about 2000 children. The day care centres are for children and youth with all types of mental disability and behavioural problems. They cannot even meet 10% of the demand in each region – usually one centre has a capacity of 30–40 children. They are under the authority of municipalities and are funded by the Ministry of Labour and Social Policy. Most of the activities are aimed at training in social and daily living skills, rehabilitation, speech therapy and psychological support.
- Croatia: equally available to the whole population; services seriously understaffed.
- Georgia: there is only one day treatment facility for children. Because of stigma (it is located on the grounds of the psychiatric hospital), very few children visit.
- Germany: 204 day treatment facilities for young people with disabilities and 8038 youth centres.
- Greece: there is only one day centre for mentally ill children in Athens.
- Ireland: currently there are 45 child and adolescent mental health teams, with 585 team members, providing clinical interventions on a day treatment basis.

Social institutions

Social institutions for children and adolescents are provided in 31 of 42 countries (74%), in comparable proportions across the groups of countries. This is the area with the largest variation in care. In countries in western Europe, children are often placed in foster homes or small residential facilities. In many countries in south-eastern Europe and CIS countries, children with any form of disability are placed in sometimes large and often underfunded social care homes. Some of the descriptions below give a flavour.

- Azerbaijan: there are two social institutions for children with severe mental disability and six boarding schools; a program of deinstitutionalization has started, and social institutions will be closed or transformed by 2015.
- Bosnia and Herzegovina (Federation of Bosnia and Herzegovina): there are two residential institutions covering the needs of children disabled in general, including mental retardation and long-term mental disorder.
- Bulgaria: 27 homes with about 1200 children and 428 adolescents. These homes are in extremely poor condition compared with other institutions and community-

Table 6.20. Availability of specialized mental health services for children and adolescents in various types of facilities in groups of countries

Facilities with specialized services for children and adolescents	EU		EU15		New EU countries since 2004		Israel, Norway and Switzerland		South-eastern Europe		CIS		Total	
	No.	%	No.	%	No.	%	No.	%	No.	%	No.	%	No.	%
Mental hospitals														
Yes	19	70	9	60	10	83	2	67	5	71	4	80	30	71
No	6	22	5	33	1	8	0	0	1	14	1	20	8	19
Information not available	2	7	1	7	1	8	1	33	1	14	0	0	4	10
Community-based psychiatric inpatient units and units in district general hospitals														
Yes	19	70	14	93	5	42	3	100	3	43	2	40	27	64
No	7	26	1	7	6	50	0	0	3	43	3	60	13	31
Information not available	1	4	0	0	1	8	0	0	1	14	0	0	2	5
Mental health outpatient facilities														
Yes	26	96	15	100	11	92	3	100	6	86	5	100	40	95
No	1	4	0	0	1	8	0	0	0	0	0	0	1	2
Information not available	0	0	0	0	0	0	0	0	1	14	0	0	1	2
Day treatment facilities														
Yes	22	81	14	93	8	67	3	100	3	43	4	80	32	76
No	4	15	1	7	3	25	0	0	3	43	1	20	8	19
Information not available	1	4	0	0	1	8	0	0	1	14	0	0	2	5
Residential facilities that are not health care (social institutions)														
Yes	21	78	12	80	9	75	1	33	4	57	5	100	31	74
No	3	11	1	7	2	17	1	33	1	14	0	0	5	12
Information not available	3	11	2	13	1	8	1	33	2	29	0	0	6	14

based services for children. The level of care is very low and the children are largely neglected.

- Georgia: there are two state orphanages in Kaspi and Senaki for disabled children and six boarding schools for children with intellectual and physical disability (14.7 per 100 000 population). In these institutions the conditions are appalling.
- Germany: 2354 residential places to support raising children, including nongovernmental organizations.

Main activities initiated and developed since 2005 related to the mental health of children and adolescents

- Finland: (1) Intergenerational transfer of mental disorder and social exclusion is a major societal problem. Services have therefore been developed in the national health care system for children and families in which the parents have a mental disorder. (2) School is a major context for children's social and emotional development. A programme was initiated in 2006 to develop interventions for teachers to promote children's development in the school setting. The interventions will be implemented countrywide. (3) Health promotion activities, including mental health, are being mapped countrywide in health services and in the school system to provide a basis for further development.
- France: the Psychiatry and Mental Health Plan 2005–2008 supports the development of 75 homes for adolescents in France between 2005 and 2010. A national action programme for family doctors in training the recognition of children and adolescents with mental disorders has been delivered.
- Ireland: 16 additional child and adolescent mental health teams will be recruited in 2006 and 2007. Additional inpatient places will be available later in 2007.

- Lithuania: child and adolescent health is one of the mental health priorities that will be supported by the EU Structural Funds in 2007–2013.
- Malta: a programme for the early detection and management of depression among schoolchildren. A joint committee between the Ministry of Health and Ministry of Social Solidarity and the Family carried out a review on the services available for children and adolescents. The objective is to provide a holistic and seamless service to this client group.
- United Kingdom (England and Wales): a selection of relevant activities are:
  - 2005: government sponsorship of the National CAMHS Support Service, a service improvement team working with local partnerships to improve the commissioning and delivery of a comprehensive range of services that are culturally competent and easy to access.
  - 2005: joint health and local authority performance indicators relating to learning disability, services for 16- to 17-year-olds and 24/7 availability and provision for children with complex levels of need.
  - 2005: development of a cultural competence tool for local teams and leaflets for children, adolescents and parents in 14 languages explaining "What are mental health services for children and adolescents?".
  - Publication of National Institute for Health and Clinical Excellence guidelines on teenage depression, self-harm, eating disorders, attention deficit hyperactivity syndrome and parenting.
  - Development of local behaviour intervention plans in schools, ensuring coordinated support to children with challenging behaviour and behaviour intervention support teams, multidisciplinary teams targeting vulnerable children.
- Uzbekistan: an "infant psychiatry" service was created with the purpose of early detection and health improvement for children aged 0–4 years with mental and nervous system disorders; it functions in coordination with maternity hospitals, departments of newborn pathology and child treatment and prophylactic institutions. This service is working in most regions. At the beginning of 2007, the "infant psychiatry" service observed 1590 children, 83 children were taken under observation and 281 were taken off the observation during the first quarter of 2007.

Mental health services for older people

This section provides information about the presence of specialized mental health services for older people (Table 6.21). The survey enquired about available services in inpatient, outpatient and residential settings. Capacity, conditions and staffing levels vary again between countries, and some of the examples illustrate this.

Inpatient facilities

Mental hospitals

Almost seventy per cent of the countries have specialized mental health care for older people in mental hospitals. In most of these countries mental hospitals have separate departments for older people.

- Czech Republic: specialized geriatric departments within a mental hospital.
- Georgia: older people are treated in the psychiatric hospitals. There is no specialized geriatric unit in the country.
- Latvia: each mental hospital has separate departments for old people with mental problems – mostly dementia. These departments are called somato-geriatric departments (such as dementia or dementia plus somatic problems).
- Ireland: a few older adults continue to reside in traditional psychiatric hospitals. The current national policy is to close large psychiatric hospitals, and it is planned that these adults will move in to more appropriate community-based residential facilities.
- Switzerland: integrated into existing institutions (geriatric or geriatric psychiatry departments in hospitals, dementia groups in care homes etc.).

Table 6.21. Availability of specialized mental health services for older people in various types of facilities in groups of countries

Facilities with specialized services for older people	EU		EU15		New EU countries since 2004		Israel, Norway and Switzerland		South-eastern Europe		CIS		Total	
	No.	%	No.	%	No.	%	No.	%	No.	%	No.	%	No.	%
Mental hospitals														
Yes	18	67	10	67	8	67	3	100	4	57	4	80	29	69
No	7	26	3	20	4	33	0	0	3	43	1	20	11	26
Information not available	2	7	2	13	0	0	0	0	0	0	0	0	2	5
Community-based psychiatric inpatient units and units in district general hospitals														
Yes	12	44	7	47	5	42	3	100	2	29	2	40	19	45
No	13	48	6	40	7	58	0	0	5	71	3	60	21	50
Information not available	2	7	2	13	0	0	0	0	0	0	0	0	2	5
Mental health outpatient facilities														
Yes	15	56	11	73	4	33	2	67	4	57	4	80	25	60
No	9	33	1	7	8	67	0	0	3	43	1	20	13	31
Information not available	3	11	3	20	0	0	1	33	0	0	0	0	4	10
Day treatment facilities														
Yes	18	67	11	73	7	58	2	67	2	29	3	60	25	60
No	5	19	0	0	5	42	1	33	5	71	2	40	13	31
Information not available	4	15	4	27	0	0	0	0	0	0	0	0	4	10
Residential facilities that are not health care (social institutions)														
Yes	17	63	10	67	7	58	1	33	4	57	5	100	27	64
No	4	15	0	0	4	33	1	33	1	14	0	0	6	14
Information not available	6	22	5	33	1	8	1	33	2	29	0	0	9	21
Community residential health facilities														
Yes	8	30	7	47	1	8	1	33	3	43	2	40	14	33
No	14	52	5	33	9	75	1	33	4	57	3	60	22	52
Information not available	5	19	3	20	2	17	1	33	0	0	0	0	6	14

Community-based psychiatric inpatient units and units in district general hospitals

Community-based psychiatric inpatient units and units in district general hospitals for older people are available in 19 of 42 countries (45%), mostly in EU countries.

- Czech Republic: 10 acute geriatric care departments with 545 beds.
- Ireland: there are 62 acute designated assessment and treatment beds, some in specially designated locations within acute general hospital units.
- Lithuania: not specialized for older people but available in common psychiatric departments.

Outpatient facilities

Mental health outpatient facilities

Specialized mental health outpatient facilities for older people are available in 25 of 42 countries (60%) but can vary greatly in functioning.

- Austria: two facilities in Vienna and two in Styria.
- Denmark: dementia teams for home treatment.
- Hungary: "dementia centres" covering the whole country. Both neurological and psychiatric facilities are accredited as "centres".
- Ireland: there are 20 consultant-supported specialist mental health teams for older people. A total of 42 teams is required to provide one specialist team per 100 000 of

the population. Existing specialist teams provide outpatient treatment interventions through centralized review clinics and home-based assessments.

- Lithuania: help for older people is available in mental health centres, but there are no specialized services.
- Russian Federation: establishment of specialized geriatric psychiatry rooms has been elaborated and soon will be introduced into practice all over the country.
- Serbia: a specialized outpatient facility for older people was opened at the Institute for Mental Health in 2007, with home treatment when needed. The club for the third age started in February 2008.

Day treatment facilities

Day treatment facilities are available for older people in 25 of 42 countries (60%), slightly more in the EU15 countries (73%).

- Hungary: in the social sector a new type of day care has been developed for people with dementia.
- Italy: 560 specialized centres for dementia.
- Lithuania: there is only one psychosocial specialized centre in Vilnius for people with Alzheimer disease and other age-related disorders.
- Spain (Catalonia): day centres for older people.
- Spain (Extremadura): day centres for people with Alzheimer disease (Centros de Día para Alzheimer).
- Switzerland: in large psychiatric centres (such as in Basle) there are geriatric psychiatry day hospitals and outpatient clinics etc. "Memory clinics" offer specific explanations and sometimes special cognitive training.

Social institutions

Social institutions are available in 27 of 42 countries (64%). The high proportion (100%) of institutions in CIS countries represents social care homes, as described by Georgia. The differences in the quality of care compared with such countries as Austria and Italy can be striking.

- Austria: old people with mental disorders are mainly in non-specialized residential facilities.
- Georgia: there are no specialized residential facilities for old people with mental disorders; they are mainly provided care by social institutions with poor conditions.
- Italy: when mental hospitals were closed, the older people with minor psychiatric diagnoses were moved to small social residential facilities already in existence or newly established.
- Uzbekistan: "mercy homes" are functioning within the system of the Ministry of Labor and Social Security, in which war veterans, lonely pensioners and people with disability are living. Seven additional sanatoriums and boarding houses are provided for this population group.

Access to interventions

Access to psychosocial interventions

The survey enquired about the proportion of service users who received one or more psychosocial interventions in the last available year in different facilities. The questionnaire asked about such interventions in outpatient facilities, day treatment facilities, community-based psychiatric inpatient units and mental hospitals.

Half the countries consistently replied that this information was not available. The answers received were based on estimates and on impressions of how services functioned rather than data collected through an information system. The country examples below illustrate this. The many countries commenting that data were not available are omitted.

- Azerbaijan: psychosocial interventions are not available in the country.
- Denmark: there are no data, but usually most severe or chronic service users will receive some psychosocial intervention as part of the mental health service, such as a sheltered workplace, pension support etc.

Definition

Psychosocial interventions are defined as interventions using primarily psychological or social methods for treating and/or rehabilitating a person with a mental disorder or substantial reducing their psychosocial distress.

Psychosocial interventions include: psychotherapy; counselling; activities with families; psychoeducational treatments; providing social support; rehabilitation activities (such as leisure and socializing activities, interpersonal and social skills training, occupational activities, vocational training and sheltered employment activities).

Psychosocial interventions exclude: intake interviews; assessment; and follow-up pharmaceutical appointments as psychosocial interventions.

Psychosocial intervention sessions should last a minimum of 20 minutes to be counted for this item. Examples of psychosocial treatment include psychotherapy, providing social support, counselling, rehabilitation activities, interpersonal and social skills training and psychoeducational treatment. They do not include intake interviews, assessment and follow-up pharmaceutical appointments.

- France: the multidisciplinary teams practising in the mental health services have a mission of social inclusion for all the users of services, performed together with the community services. The various interventions are not quantified.
- Italy: precise data can only be gathered at the regional level.
- Netherlands: most settings offer psychosocial interventions besides psychiatric care.
- Switzerland: initial statistical results from the Obsan project on outpatient and partial inpatient psychiatric services in Switzerland should be available in the second half of 2008.
- United Kingdom (Scotland): information is not readily available centrally. Delivering for mental health includes a focus on increasing access to psychological interventions in a range of settings.

Use of prescribed antidepressants

The survey enquired about the proportion of the population that had been prescribed antidepressants in the last year available (Table 6.22). Many countries (26 of 42) reported that they had no information available. Further, data on prescribed antidepressants are not collected consistently.

Table 6.22. Proportion of the population prescribed antidepressants in countries, last year available

Country	Population prescribed antidepressants (%)
Moldova	12
Spain (Catalonia)	9.8
Denmark	7
Belgium	6.1
Norway	6
Spain (Extremadura)	5.5
Hungary	5.2
Slovenia	3.3
Lithuania	3
Bosnia and Herzegovina (Republika Srpska)	1.1

For the countries who were able to submit the requested information, the proportion of the population prescribed antidepressants varied from 12% in Moldova and 10% in Spain (Catalonia) to 3% in Lithuania and 1% in Bosnia and Herzegovina (Republika Srpska).

- Belgium: 6.1% of the population (15 years and older) took prescribed antidepressants in the two weeks before the interview (data from the Health Interview Survey 2004).
- Bosnia and Herzegovina (Republika Srpska): for antidepressants, the number of medications given on prescriptions (on the positive list of the Health Insurance Fund of Republika Srpska) (data for 2006).

- Lithuania: data according to self-report in health survey provided by Statistics Lithuania.
- Moldova: the reason given for the high proportion of people prescribed antidepressants is that they can be prescribed not only by psychiatrists but also by other physicians such as cardiologists and neurologists.

Several other countries provided information on the defined daily doses (DDD) of antidepressants.

- Estonia: 13.2 DDD per 1000 population.
- Italy: 66 DDD per 1000 population.
- Sweden: 70 DDD per 1000 population.

Other countries provided yet other forms of information.

- In Austria, 3 763 000 prescriptions were written, or 0.45 prescriptions per person.
- In Germany, the per capita consumption was 0.25 packages.
- In Switzerland, the only figure available is expenditure on antidepressants as a share of total expenditure on pharmaceuticals based on out-of-factory prices (3.8%).
- In the United Kingdom (England and Wales), 31 million prescriptions were issued for antidepressants in 2006 (0.6 per person). The Office for National Statistics estimated that, in 1998, GPs treated 75.5 cases of depression per 1000 patients for women and 30.6 for men, but treatment is not specified.

Sex distribution

Sex distribution of visits and admissions

Only about half the countries provided information on the distribution of visits and admissions by male and female service users (Table 6.23). Many countries report that these data are not available. Only in Azerbaijan and Italy was the proportion of visits among men in outpatient visits higher than among women, and in all countries except for Italy the proportion of male users was higher in inpatient facilities than in outpatient facilities. Many countries had more male than female admissions to inpatient beds, but this was not consistent.

Sex distribution of beds and places

Most countries could not provide information on the distribution of beds and places by the sex of the residents. Often the reason for this was that beds were not categorized by sex to allow flexibility in occupancy. This raises the question of how beds are allocated in countries with more than one bed to a room, as is the situation in most countries, compared with countries with mostly single-bed rooms such as Denmark. In practice, the experience is that rooms, if not wards, are mostly separated by sex.

A representative sample of comments is as follows.

- Austria: not available because the wards are mixed in many settings.
- Belgium: beds and places are not specifically provided for men or women.
- Bosnia and Herzegovina (Republika Srpska): the proportion of male and female beds is 45% for both. The other 10% is flexible and depends on current needs.
- Croatia: only the total number of beds is available; information on the proportion of female and male users is not available.
- Czech Republic: information about beds for men and women in psychiatric departments in general hospitals and mental hospitals is not available.
- Denmark: beds not registered by sex. Usually beds can be used flexibly depending on need – units in general have a mix of both men and women – as most of the beds are single-bed rooms.
- Finland: almost all wards are mixed, meaning that there is no such thing as a "male bed" or "female bed".

Access to and appropriateness of mental health services for linguistic and ethnic minorities and other vulnerable groups

Access to mental health services for linguistic minorities

Countries were asked to indicate whether mental health facilities have a specific strategy to ensure that linguistic minorities can access mental health services in the language in which they are fluent (Table 6.24).

Table 6.23. Visits to mental health outpatient facilities and admissions to inpatient units (combination of community-based psychiatric inpatient units, units in district general hospitals and mental hospitals) according to sex in countries

Country	Visits to mental health outpatient facilities		Admissions to inpatient units	
	Male users (%)	Female users (%)	Male users (%)	Female users (%)
Austria	Information not available	Information not available	51	49
Azerbaijan	75	25	Information not available	Information not available
Belgium	Information not available	Information not available	51	49
Bosnia and Herzegovina (Republika Srpska)	Information not available	Information not available	67	33
Czech Republic	41	59	54	46
Denmark	44	56	48	52
Estonia	Information not available	Information not available	43	57
Finland	Information not available	Information not available	50	50
Germany	Information not available	Information not available	54	46
Hungary	33	67	45	55
Ireland	Information not available	Information not available	51	49
Israel	Information not available	Information not available	58	42
Italy	58	42	50	50
Latvia	45	55	48	52
Malta	Information not available	Information not available	65	35
Moldova	37	63	45	55
Spain				
Castilla y Léon	40	60	52	48
Catalonia	41	59	Information not available	Information not available
Galicia	36	64	56	44
Sweden	40	60	60	40
The former Yugoslav Republic of Macedonia	45	55	60	40
United Kingdom				
England and Wales	45	55	50	50
Scotland	47	52	50	49

Many countries have not addressed access to mental health services in a language appropriate to minorities. Few countries in the region (Norway, Slovenia and the United Kingdom (England and Wales)) report having specific strategies in place in all or almost all mental health facilities to ensure that linguistic minorities can access mental health services in the language in which they are fluent.

In more than 40% of the countries such strategies are not present in any facility, and in 12 of the 42 countries (29%), strategies are present in less than 20% of the mental health facilities.

In some of the countries that indicate that such strategies exist, both the main population and minority groups, including service users and health professionals, are fluent in the relevant languages (such as Russian and the national languages of Azerbaijan, Estonia and Lithuania). Many very similar comments are summarized below.

- Azerbaijan: there are mental health services in two languages (Azerbaijani and Russian). All minorities speak at least one of them, and all or almost all of the population can therefore access mental health services in the language in which they are fluent.

- Bosnia and Herzegovina (Federation of Bosnia and Herzegovina): there are no specific language minorities in numbers to require mental health services in their language. The Roma population is the largest minority, but they speak the national language.
- Estonia: linguistic problems are solved on an ad hoc basis. The biggest minority in Estonia is Russian-speaking people, and health care personnel can communicate without problems in Russian.

For diverse groups of immigrants and minorities, offering access in a language in which they are fluent has been identified as a problem, particularly in countries with a large number of immigrants and minorities. Some of these countries, mostly in western Europe, have developed diverse strategies:

- Austria: two intercultural outpatient clinics, one at the Department of Psychiatry and Psychotherapy of the Medical University of Vienna and one at the Wagner Jauregg Nervenklinik in Linz.
- Denmark: there is a legal right to have a translator when needed, including for deaf people. There is a unit with Greenlandic-speaking staff.
- Finland: the lack of special services for linguistic minorities constitutes a barrier to access to mental health services. Some special services for Swedish-speaking people exist in Helsinki.
- France: the mental health services can rely on associations providing interpreting services to the linguistic minorities as well as services specializing in ethnic psychiatry and cultural mediation.
- Germany: in recent years diverse and innovative projects have been launched and have markedly improved the situation regarding communication and cultural understanding.
  - A successful approach was realized in Lower Saxony. The Ministry for Social, Women's and Family Affairs funds a health service that plays a moderating, networking, intercultural role, the Ethno-Medical Centre (Ethno-Medizinisches Zentrum) in Hanover. Public social and health services in the region of Hanover can request interpreters when needed. The Centre is now establishing a similar service in Munich in cooperation with the Bavarian Centre for Transcultural Medicine (Bayerisches Zentrum für Transkulturelle Medizin e.V.). The 200 interpreters who work for

Table 6.24. Mental health facilities using a specific strategy to ensure that linguistic minorities can access mental health services in the language in which they are fluent in groups of countries

Mental health facilities with specific strategies for linguistic minorities	EU		EU15		New EU countries since 2004		Israel, Norway and Switzerland		South-eastern Europe		CIS		Total	
	No.	%	No.	%	No.	%	No.	%	No.	%	No.	%	No.	%
Have a strategy														
Yes	16	59	14	93	2	17	3	100	3	43	2	40	24	57
No	10	37	1	7	9	75	0	0	4	57	3	60	17	40
Information not available	1	4	0	0	1	8	0	0	0	0	0	0	1	2
Proportion using a strategy														
All or almost all (81–100%)	2	7	1	7	1	8	1	33	0	0	0	0	3	7
Majority (51–80%)	2	7	2	13	0	0	0	0	1	14	1	20	4	10
Some (21–50%)	4	15	4	27	0	0	1	33	0	0	0	0	5	12
A few (1–20%)	8	30	7	47	1	8	1	33	2	29	1	20	12	29
None	10	37	1	7	9	75	0	0	4	57	3	60	17	41
Information not available	1	4	0	0	1	8	0	0	0	0	0	0	1	2

the Community Interpreter Service in Hanover and Munich cover a range of 50 languages. In both centres the referral service sends trained interpreters, and evaluates their performance. The Ethno-Medical Centre is also currently supporting the establishment of a local Community Interpreter Service Berlin (Gemeindedolmetschdienst Berlin) within the framework of an EQUAL Project funded by the European Social Fund conducted by Berlin Health (Gesundheit Berlin e.V.). Currently, an extensive curriculum is being implemented here, and roughly 50 people – people who are unemployed and people who are receiving social assistance who have extensive linguistic skills – are being trained in a one-year course to be deployed as community interpreters according to the models in Hanover and Munich. The Community Interpreter Service employs people with migrant status who have been trained in social communication as a "bridge between cultures". Their task is to facilitate linguistic and cultural understanding and effective help between the social services and health care systems and migrants.
- The director of the interface project Hamburg/Schnelsen, Joachim Gerbing, developed a neighbourhood-oriented interpreter service, employing voluntary community interpreters. Voluntary community interpreters are trained to establish a uniform standard for interpreters, who are mainly employed to provide social support. They accompany clients on doctors' and lawyers' visits.
- An interim interpreter service was established in Frankfurt to translate over the telephone. However, this service was discontinued since it was not used often enough.
- In many cities the idea of promoting health care through better linguistic networking has also emerged. In Cologne and Frankfurt, for example, directories of multilingual doctors and health facilities with multilingual personnel were compiled.
- The funding of outpatient interpreter services in connection with medical and psychotherapy services is still a problem. The health care funds do not pay for these services on an outpatient basis. The reason cited is that the health care funds can only pay for services that are provided under the responsibility of doctors, and this is not the case for interpreter services. For inpatient care, the hospitals finance interpreter services from their overall budget.

- Ireland: almost 10% of the residents in Ireland are non-Irish nationals. Most of these are young people (62%) and single (68%). Formal policy within the specialist mental health service is to ensure, as far as possible, that linguistic minorities can access mental health services in their own language. This would be (and is) done on an interpretation service basis as the need arises. Of interest, 62% of non-consultant hospital doctors in Ireland's mental health system are foreign nationals, and many psychiatric nurses have been recruited from outside the EU. A vision for change notes that good communication is at the heart of mental health work. The question of language is therefore extremely important. Good interpreters are vital not just for effective cross-cultural working but also for ensuring access to mental health services by other individuals in the population, specifically deaf individuals and those for whom Irish is their first language. Mental health work requires interpreters who are able to interpret the idiom of the patient's distress as well as the actual words used. Interpreters must be able to empathize with the patient's position, and ethnic and gender conflicts are to be avoided. Further, the Official Languages Act of 2003 may place additional responsibilities on health services in relation to services to the Irish-speaking population.
- Israel: local initiatives of a few units.
- Netherlands: there are special programmes to provide care for the different minorities within the programmes of several organizations across the country. These mental health organizations have special units for providing care to asylum-seekers

and some of them for minorities such as Surinamese, Antillean and Moroccan immigrants.

- Serbia: there are many ethnic minorities, but they all speak Serbian. Various nongovernmental organizations have developed a few psychosocial programmes for Roma people.
- Slovenia: Italian and Hungarian minorities can speak in their own language since doctors employed in the bilingual areas need to pass the exam in both languages and use it fluently.
- Switzerland: according to health monitoring of Switzerland's migrant population, a high proportion of those questioned in the Swiss Health Survey 2002 achieve communication in one of Switzerland's national languages. The use of translation assistance varies considerably with language knowledge in the relevant groups. According to information from those questioned, language mediation from professional translators or interpreters has not been available to any appreciable extent so far. Relatives (such as spouses or children) are of paramount importance. The availability and quality of language mediation varies from institution to institution. The institutions themselves bear the cost of professional language mediation. The joint project Migrant Friendly Hospitals – a hospital network for the migrant population of the Federal Office of Public Health and the Swiss Hospital Association aims to create a network of hospitals, psychiatric clinics, rehabilitation clinics and long-term care institutions that are characterized by special competence in the care of the migrant population.

Use of mental health services by ethnic and minority groups

A challenge in many countries is providing equitable use of mental health services by ethnic and minority groups. An indicator is whether this is proportionate in comparison to their relative population size.

Most countries have difficulty reporting on the proportion of ethnic and minority groups that use outpatient mental health services (19 of 42 countries) and mental hospitals (22 of 42 countries) compared with their relative proportion of the population (Table 6.25). Some countries indicate that they cannot provide information since no assessments had been performed. Other countries informed us that answers are estimates.

In countries for which this information is available, the following can be noted.

Table 6.25. Use of mental health services by ethnic and minority groups compared with their relative population size in groups of countries

Representation of groups in use of mental health services	EU		EU15		New EU countries since 2004		Israel, Norway and Switzerland		South-eastern Europe		CIS		Total	
	No.	%	No.	%	No.	%	No.	%	No.	%	No.	%	No.	%
Outpatient services														
Equally represented	4	15	1	7	3	25	0	0	5	71	2	40	11	26
Substantially underrepresented	10	37	10	67	0	0	0	0	0	0	1	20	11	26
Substantially overrepresented	1	4	0	0	1	8	0	0	0	0	0	0	1	2
Information not available	12	44	4	27	8	67	3	100	2	29	2	40	19	45
Mental hospitals														
Equally represented	8	30	5	33	3	25	0	0	4	57	3	60	15	36
Substantially underrepresented	2	7	2	13	0	0	1	33	0	0	0	0	3	7
Substantially overrepresented	2	7	1	7	1	8	0	0	0	0	0	0	2	5
Information not available	15	56	7	47	8	67	2	67	3	43	2	40	22	52

- In outpatient services, service users from ethnic and minority groups are almost equally represented in 26% of the countries (11 of 42). They are substantially underrepresented in 26% of the countries (11 of 42). This includes 10 of the EU15 countries and the Russian Federation.
- In hospitals, 36% of the countries (15 of 42) report equal representation. Only the United Kingdom (England and Wales) and Estonia report that they are substantially overrepresented. Belgium, Greece and Switzerland report substantial underrepresentation in mental hospitals.

Some of the countries do not record the ethnicity of service users on admission. It was also mentioned that the Roma population tends to access mental health services less frequently, as many are not insured.

- Belgium: not everyone finds the way to the appropriate care due to difficulty owing to cultural differences. For suicide attempts, the proportion of immigrants versus locals that are reported is higher in hospital emergency services than in GP offices.
- Bosnia and Herzegovina (Federation of Bosnia and Herzegovina): they have rights to equal access to all services as the majority population in the country. But due to the economic and social status of the Roma population, they visit mental health services less than other people do. Many are not covered by health insurance.
- Bulgaria: substantially underrepresented in social care homes for mentally disabled adults. Substantially overrepresented in special schools for children with intellectual disability.
- Denmark: overrepresented in forensic units and underrepresented in outpatient and ordinary inpatient services.
- Switzerland: the number of discharges of people older than 14 years in inpatient institutions- total number 52 800; number of Swiss nationals 52 100 (99%); number of non-Swiss nationals 700 (1%). Given that non-Swiss nationals comprise 21% of the population, they are clearly underrepresented.

Discussion

Mental health services cover a large number of service components, and this chapter has presented many of these. Many of the tables show the variation in attendance, numbers and distribution of beds, number of admissions, duration of stay, availability of community services and, for a few countries, prescribing patterns.

Some discussion points arise. Two very different clusters of countries have the fewest beds. The first seems to group countries with low level of investment in mental health care and low supply of services such as Albania, Turkey and possibly Portugal. The second group, comprising Italy, some provinces in Spain and the United Kingdom (England and Wales), are in the post-hospital stage, having replaced beds with community services. Some countries, such as Belgium, France, Germany and the Netherlands, combine a high level of beds with community services. Whether this is the best or worst of both worlds is an important debate.

Visits to mental health facilities show a wide range of differences in access, from 1% to 28% of the population. Some of this can be explained by counting multiple visits, but considerable variation would still remain. Some countries with low rates are likely to offer alternative services, either by primary care or community teams.

Admissions to inpatient units also vary significantly, from 0.1% to 1.3% of the population. At the high end are such countries as Estonia, Hungary and Romania together with such countries as Germany and Sweden. In some cases, the high admission rates could be due to perverse financial incentives within the health system such as payment per admission or payment for a limited period of admission only, encouraging discharge and readmission. In other countries, a large supply of beds could be a factor.

Intriguing is the finding of overrepresentation of women in outpatient services but almost equal sex distribution in inpatient services. This confirms earlier studies.

The lack of community service provision is not surprising, although the gap between policy and practice is striking. Possibly of greatest concern is the absence of provision for 24-hour crisis services in many countries.

Data on access to psychosocial interventions were mostly absent. Although this is not surprising, it deserves some consideration given the growing evidence of effectiveness of some of these interventions. The difficulty in obtaining consistent prescribing data for so many countries means that any interpretation has to be cautious. However, the high rates and the variation are evident, even for the small number of countries. Compared with the rate of severe depression, about 2–4%, this shows that prescribing practices for people with depressive symptoms are very liberal in many countries. This can account for a large proportion of the mental health care budget.

The comments in the section on residential and social homes for people with mental disorders comprise a powerful argument for carefully assessing spending priorities. Conditions in some of these places, home for life of the most vulnerable people in society, as recognized by the countries, can be shocking. A slight readjustment in spending from expensive and not always effective prescription drugs to providing care could make a great difference.

Services for children and adolescents and services for older people show predictable variation. More important than these numbers is access and quality, and it is hoped that this will be addressed in the near future. Particularly long-term care for these groups can be an area of concern.

Finally, many countries are struggling to offer culture- and language-sensitive services. It is interesting that some countries report underrepresentation of admissions from minority groups and others overrepresentation. Clearly, more detailed comparison is required.

In combination, this chapter powerfully demonstrates several points.

The provision of mental health services varies tremendously across the WHO European Region. Although several countries have similar service structures, particularly in the more institutionalized part of the Region, even these countries show considerable variation in the number of beds, admissions and community care developments such as crisis services and units in district general hospitals. Services in the EU15 countries appear to be so differentiated that any comparison is haphazard.

Associated with the differentiation is the growing complexity of mental health services. An example is England, where about 10 years ago only few community teams were in existence. Now more than 700 community teams are spread around the country, many specializing in crisis services, assertive outreach, early intervention or primary care liaison. The loss of mental hospital beds has been balanced by the funding of a complex network of small-scale independent sector residential facilities serving children, adolescents, adults or old people with mental health problems. Other countries have also developed sophisticated services, but of a different character. The standard monolithic provision of psychiatric services across Europe, symbolized by the large mental hospital, has been replaced in many countries by creative local service systems. This in turn has resulted in diversity, making a comparison of quality and effectiveness complex.

The development of these mental health systems powerfully shows the pace and scale of mental health reform in the European Region. The stage of reform differs considerably, as does the detail, especially when different parts of the Region are compared, but there is a consistent movement towards community-based services and closing beds, as shown in this chapter.

It would be tempting to correlate data from across this chapter and draw inferences from numbers, rates or rank orders in tables. Variables such as number of beds, rate of admissions and median length of stay as associated with the presence of residential homes and community teams seem to show this well. However, the number of variables involved and the very different contexts in many countries, considering not only the types of specialist services but also the number of psychiatrists, role of primary care, social services and level of investment, all covered in other chapters and demonstrating considerable variation across countries, makes such a task daunting. Even more challenging is the absence of consistent outcome data, a subject covered in the chapter on information.

Despite these cautionary comments, this chapter gives a detailed overall picture of mental health services in Europe, stimulating comparison and debate. The next stage would be more in-depth qualitative comparisons between countries and learning the lessons of success and failure of development.

“The recognition of involving users and carers as good practice is positive, and it is to be hoped that countries can learn from these examples and build on them”

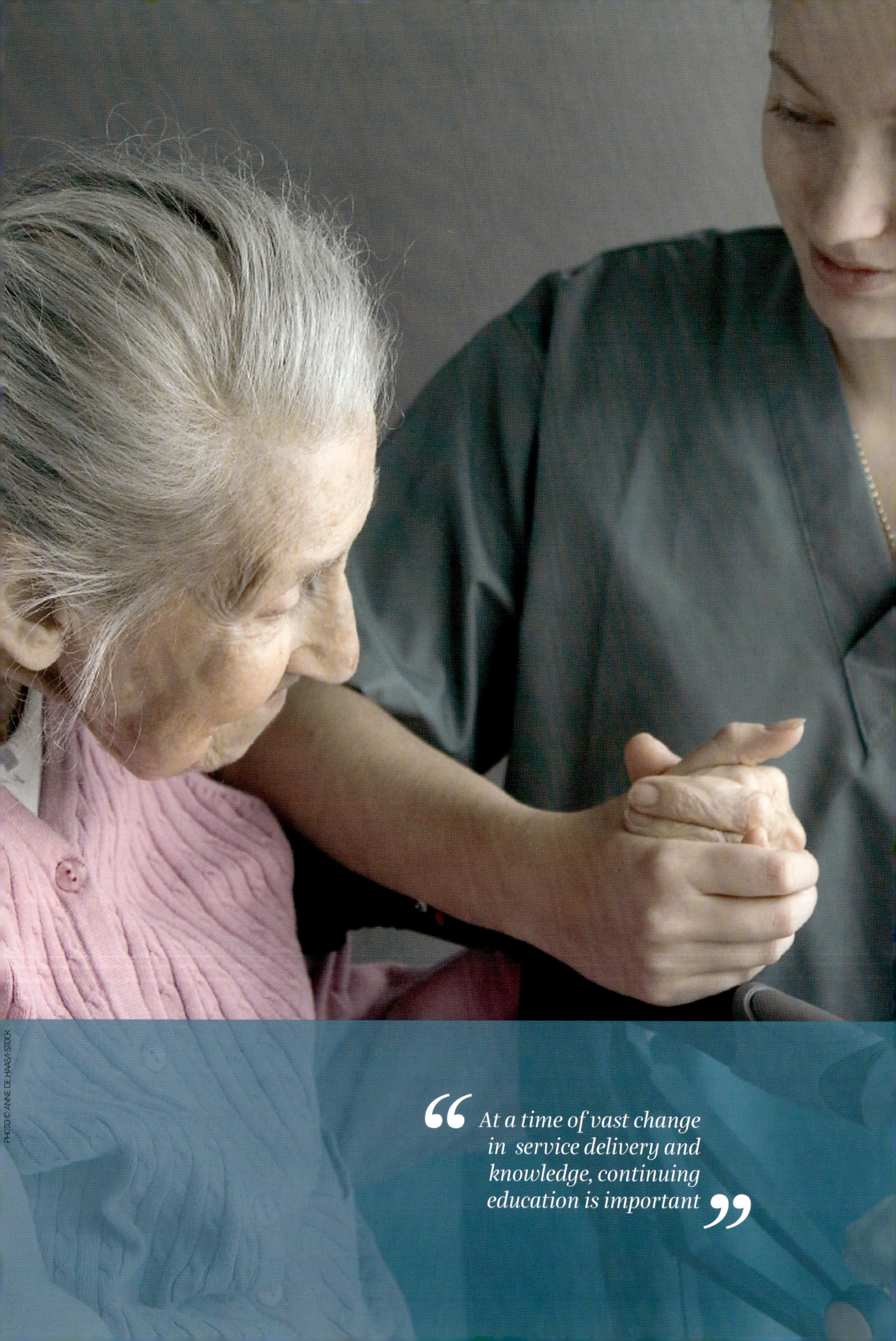

PHOTO © ANNE DE HAAS/I-STOCK

"At a time of vast change in service delivery and knowledge, continuing education is important"

7. Workforce for mental health care

Policies and services, as presented in earlier chapters, offer a vision and a structure for mental health activities. The actual delivery of interventions and the experience of the quality of care rely heavily on the workforce. Unless staff are available in sufficient numbers and are educated and trained in the required competencies, mental health services cannot operate satisfactorily and efficiently. The number and the values, attitudes and skills and knowledge of staff, in turn directly related to education and training, are central to the quality of care.

Traditionally, the mental health workforce comprised psychiatrists and nurses working in institutional settings, and this still remains the case in parts of the WHO European Region. More recently psychologists, social workers and occupational therapists entered the workforce, adding diversity, and in combination offering skills that cover identification, diagnosis, treatment, care, functional assessment, psychological therapy, psychosocial support, liaison with other agencies and rehabilitation.

Following the shift to community-based services, the staff groups have remained largely constant but roles and competencies have changed considerably. For example, the role of a doctor is very different in a traditional institutional setting compared with a community environment, where constant adjustments have to be made depending on the needs of clients and where the various staff groups that form the multidisciplinary team will be strongly mutually reliant. The role of nursing has seen even greater change in countries that have introduced community services, adjusting from reactive carers to proactive therapists, community workers and, in some cases, managers. This could be summarized as a shift from a supply-driven institutional model to a needs-led community-based system of care. A rigid and hierarchical workforce model will prove to be dysfunctional in such a complex interactive system.

This implies that reform of mental health care depends on the preparedness of staff and the opportunities they are being offered to operate effectively. The availability of numbers of personnel sufficient to deliver comprehensive interventions and care with adequate competencies to treat and support the diverse needs of people with mental health problems is a challenge that needs to be met in order to offer the benefits mental health care has proven it can deliver. Such a challenge needs to be addressed through carefully considered workforce strategies.

This chapter presents the state of the workforce in the WHO European Region, including workforce dynamics such as international migration, and highlights some of the challenges and solutions countries have developed.

National policies and programmes on the workforce for mental health care

The presence of a national workforce strategy, addressing the numbers and competencies of mental health staff to deal with the challenges of mental health development, indicates the state of reform.

Fewer than half the countries surveyed (18 of 42 countries) have such a national workforce strategy (Table 7.1). Among EU countries, 9 of the EU15 countries (60%) and only 2 of the 12 countries that joined the EU since 2004 (17%) have national workforce strategies. Four of the seven countries in south-eastern Europe report they have such strategies in

Table 7.1. Presence of national workforce policies and/or programmes in groups of countries

Workforce policies and/or programmes	EU		EU15		New EU countries since 2004		Israel, Norway and Switzerland		South-eastern Europe		CIS		Total	
	No.	%	No.	%	No.	%	No.	%	No.	%	No.	%	No.	%
Yes	11	41	9	60	2	17	2	67	4	57	1	20	18	43
No	13	48	5	33	8	67	1	33	3	43	4	80	21	50
Information not available	3	11	1	7	2	17	0	0	0	0	0	0	3	7

connection with the implementation of the South-eastern Europe Mental Health Project, which is relatively limited in scope. Moldova, also participating in the Project, is the only CIS country reporting such a strategy.

The Netherlands has no national workforce policies or programmes. However, there are many training programmes for training and higher education of the many professional groups, but these are not coordinated at the national level. At the national level only standards and competencies are prescribed and not the curricula to meet these standards.

Examples of national workforce policies and programmes include the following.

- Bosnia and Herzegovina (Republika Srpska): Education in primary health care in connection with mental health care in the community. Changing mental health curriculum for graduate and postgraduate education in mental health (students of medicine, psychiatry and psychology in the faculty for nurses, family medicine doctor, public health etc.) including a component of mental health in the community.
- Israel: Training for directors of mental health centres in hospitals and clinics.
- United Kingdom (England and Wales): In recent years, a national programme of work has been undertaken to help support the mental health workforce across health and social care. This has taken numerous forms, but primarily the focus has been on developing New Ways of Working (the NWW programme, http://newwaysofworking.org.uk), where responsibility is distributed among members of the mental health team with a move to ensure that the most advanced skills are deployed to deal with the most complex cases and the provision of supervision or support to the rest of the team; the introduction of new roles to help meet specific needs of service users and carers and to help expand the workforce; the introduction of the Creating Capable Teams Approach (CCTA) that helps mental health teams focus on the needs of service users and carers and of the capabilities that exist within the team; and the learning

Table 7.2. Number of psychiatrists per 100 000 population in countries

Country	Psychiatrists
Albania	3
Austria	13
Azerbaijan	5
Belgium	23
Bosnia and Herzegovina	
Federation of Bosnia and Herzegovina	7.4
Republika Srpska	5
Bulgaria	8.7
Croatia	8
Cyprus	6.5
Czech Republic	13.7
Denmark	11
Estonia	13
Finland	26
France	22
Georgia	5.6
Germany	8.7
Greece	15
Hungary	13.7
Ireland	7.3
Israel	8.8
Italy	9.8
Latvia	11.3
Lithuania	18
Luxembourg	Information not available
Malta	4
Moldova	6
Montenegro	6.4
Netherlands	14.5
Norway	16
Poland	5.5
Portugal	6.7
Romania	4.7
Russian Federation	10.9
Serbia	12
Slovakia	9
Slovenia	5.4
Spain	6.1
Sweden	24
Switzerland	30
The former Yugoslav Republic of Macedonia	9.5
Turkey	1
United Kingdom	
England and Wales	12.7
Scotland	10
Uzbekistan	4

and development needs of staff using the foundation of the Ten Essential Shared Capabilities framework that all staff are expected to adopt as part of their everyday practice supported by learning materials on the Ten Essential Shared Capabilities; the recovery approach; social inclusion; and race equality and cultural capability.

Availability of specialist mental health workers

Number of psychiatrists per 100 000 population

In many countries, clinical leadership and the delivery of mental health care still relies heavily on the presence of psychiatrists. The number of psychiatrists per 100 000 population ranges vary widely (Table 7.2, Fig. 7.1): from 30 per 100 000 in Switzerland and 26 in Finland to 3 in Albania and 1 in Turkey. The median rate of psychiatrists per 100 000 in the 41 countries that provided information is 9.

The median rates of psychiatrists per 100 000 population in the different parts of the WHO European Region are:

- EU15 – 12.9
- countries joining the EU since 2004 – 8.9
- countries in south-eastern Europe – 8
- CIS countries – 5.6.

Fig. 7.1. Number of psychiatrists per 100 000 population in countries

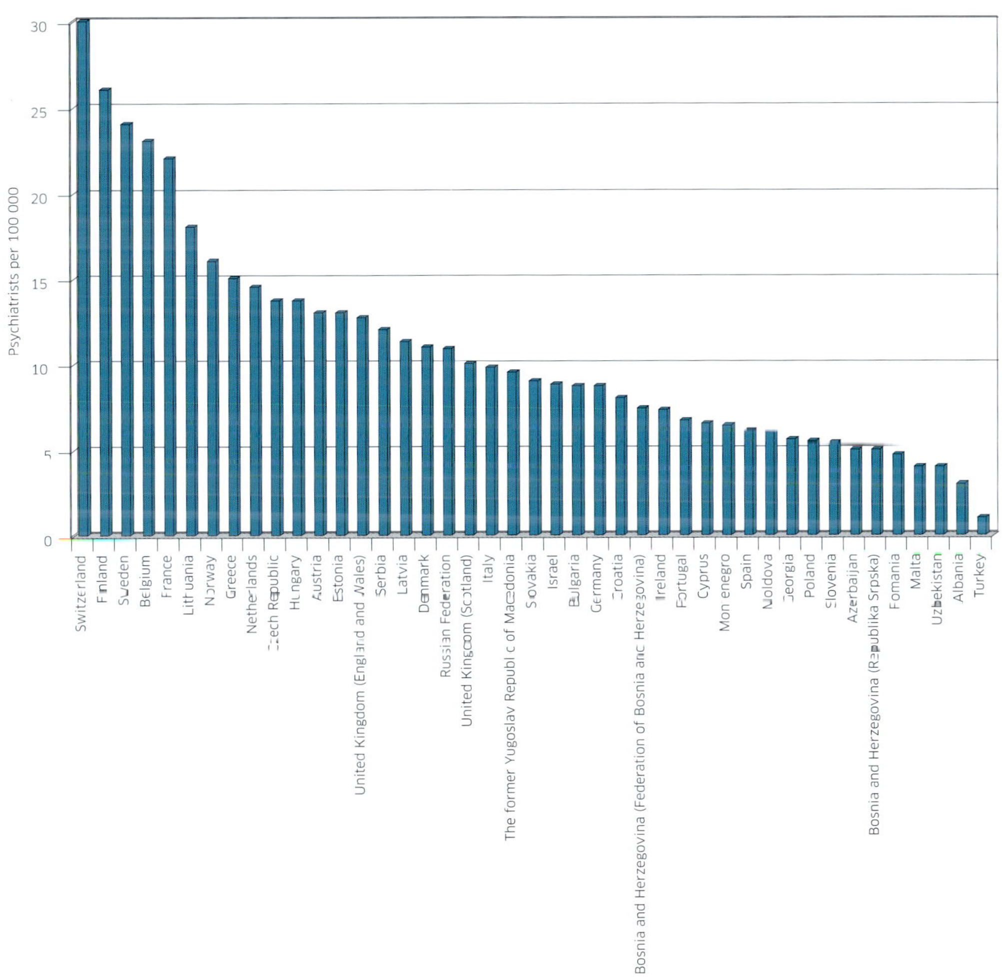

The number of psychiatrists hides differences in functions that cannot be elucidated by a survey of this kind. For example, in some countries most psychiatrists are publicly employed and work in national mental health services. In other countries psychiatrists work predominantly privately, often as psychotherapists, providing activities directly to the public or to hospitals, mostly reimbursed by insurance schemes. There are also countries with a mixed model of provision.

Number of nurses working in mental health care per 100 000 population

The shape of the frequency curve for nurses differs from that of psychiatrists (Fig. 7.2), since a few countries have a large number, whereas many have few. The rate of nurses working in mental health care varies from 163 in Finland to 4 per 100 000 population in Bosnia and Herzegovina (Republika Srpska) and 3 in Greece (Table 7.3). The median rate of nurses per 100 000 population is 21.7, more than twice the median rate of psychiatrists.

These numbers hide some important differences. Some countries offer and require a period of special training to qualify as mental health nurses, whereas others employ general nurses to work in mental health care and offer on-the-job training. Within these two categories there are further refinements.

Some countries such as Georgia note that there are no nurses trained specifically for mental health care in the country. Other countries, such as Switzerland, indicate that nurses working in mental health can have different levels of qualifications; they can have a bachelor of nursing science (three years) and master of nursing science (an additional two years); in addition master degrees in nursing science or health policy (master of public health) are offered at the university level.

Finally, some countries (such as Albania, Romania and Serbia) mix these two models. Many nurses currently working in mental health care solely have generalist training, but special courses for mental health nurses have been organized in recent years and some

Table 7.3. Number of nurses working in mental health care per 100 000 population in countries

Country	Nurses
Albania	7
Austria	37
Azerbaijan	8.4
Belgium	Information not available
Bosnia and Herzegovina	
Federation of Bosnia and Herzegovina	10
Republika Srpska	4
Bulgaria	15.5
Croatia	Information not available
Cyprus	52.5
Czech Republic	Information not available
Denmark	9
Estonia	15
Finland	163
France	Information not available
Georgia	6.7
Germany	58
Greece	3
Hungary	9.8
Ireland	126
Israel	23.4
Italy	32.9
Latvia	38
Lithuania	39
Luxembourg	Information not available
Malta	109
Moldova	14
Montenegro	Information not available
Netherlands	122
Norway	Information not available
Poland	16.4
Portugal	13.2
Romania	22.4
Russian Federation	49.7
Serbia	21
Slovenia	5.8
Slovakia	Information not available
Spain	9
Sweden	73
Switzerland	Information not available
The former Yugoslav Republic of Macedonia	24
Turkey	Information not available
United Kingdom	
England and Wales	51.9
Scotland	122
Uzbekistan	9

Fig. 7.2. Number of nurses working in mental health care per 100 000 population in countries

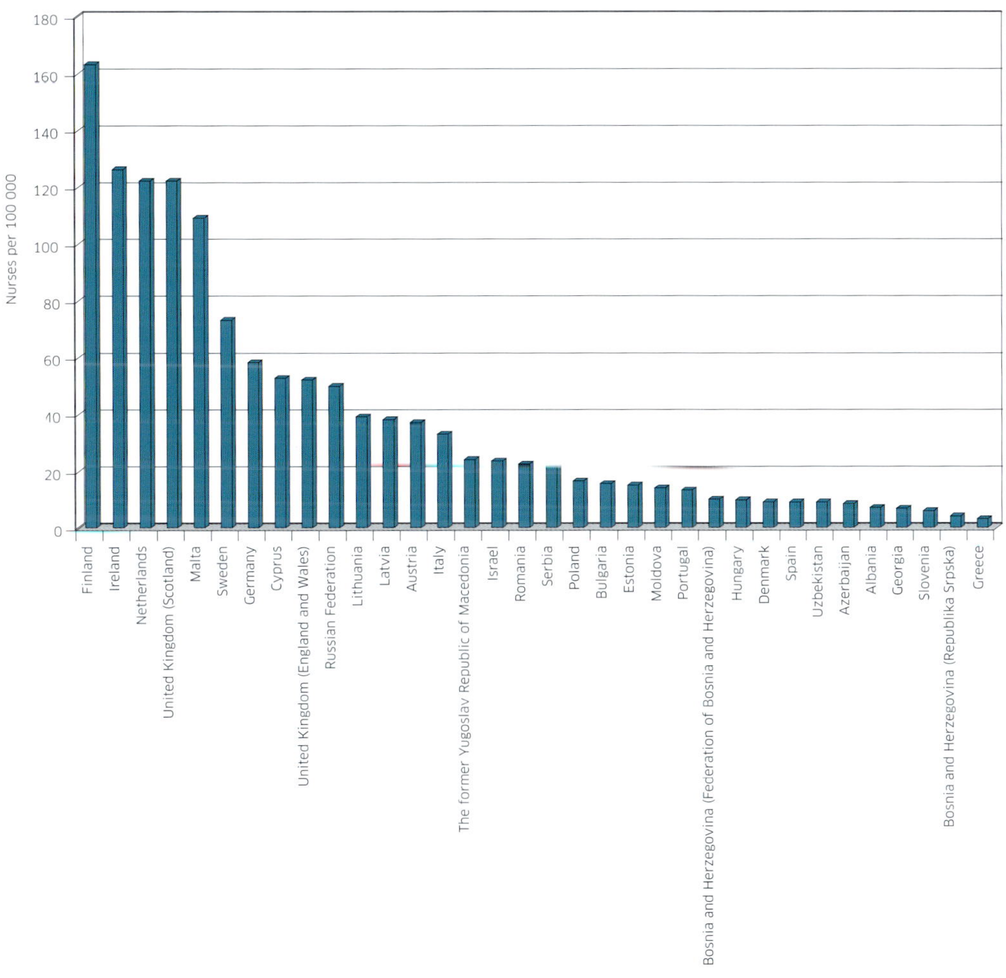

mental health nurses have already entered the workforce.

Not included in these numbers is that auxiliaries (untrained care staff) also provide additional nursing care in many countries.

Other personnel groups

Although this survey enquired about number of other staff, countries encountered major difficulty in specifying the numbers of psychologists, and even more so for social workers and occupational therapists. Table 7.4 presents information on the numbers of psychologists.

There were two challenges in specifying numbers for all these groups.

1. These staff groups functioned in generic ways in many countries, often employed by local or private agencies or institutions, and are not registered as being active in mental health care.
2. In many countries, especially CIS countries, social workers, occupational therapists and sometimes psychologists have only been established very recently, and the numbers are therefore very low.

Table 7.4. Number of psychologists working in mental health care per 100 000 population in countries

Country	Psychologists
Albania	0.5
Austria	63
Azerbaijan	0
Belgium	Information not available
Bosnia and Herzegovina	
Federation of Bosnia and Herzegovina	0.5
Republika Srpska	3
Bulgaria	0.8
Croatia	Information not available
Cyprus	6.7
Czech Republic	Information not available
Denmark	10
Estonia	Information not available
Finland	47.2
France	Information not available
Georgia	0.98
Germany	Information not available
Greece	14
Hungary	6
Ireland	Information not available
Israel	10.6
Italy	3.2
Latvia	1
Lithuania	7
Luxembourg	Information not available
Malta	6
Moldova	Information not available
Montenegro	1.5
Netherlands	30
Norway	35
Poland	4.9
Portugal	2.3
Romania	Information not available
Russian Federation	2.4
Serbia	2
Slovakia	3
Slovenia	1.7
Spain	4
Sweden	Information not available
Switzerland	Information not available
The former Yugoslav Republic of Macedonia	2
Turkey	Information not available
United Kingdom	
England and Wales	4.3
Scotland	3
Uzbekistan	1

Psychiatrists emigrating and immigrating across the European Region

Mental health reform creates a great demand for increasing the workforce. One mechanism is to attract personnel from elsewhere, either from inside or outside Europe. Many countries are concerned about the consequences of workforce migration, since they have invested considerable public money in training and since replacement can be very challenging.

The large majority of countries (35 of 42) do not have information available on the number and percentage of psychiatrists who have emigrated to other countries. The countries that do have information available report a relatively low percentage of psychiatrists emigrating, except for Moldova. Estonia reports that joining the EU has increased the emigration of doctors However, many of the countries that are known to experience emigration did not provide data. The countries reporting data on emigration are:

- Albania: 1%
- Estonia: 2%
- Georgia: 4%
- Malta and Spain (Murcia): 0%
- Moldova: 20%
- The former Yugoslav Republic of Macedonia: about 2%.

Information on the percentage of all psychiatrists who immigrated to European countries is also not available for about 80% of the countries. Of the eight countries that provided information, four (Georgia, Malta, Moldova and the former Yugoslav Republic of Macedonia) indicated that no psychiatrists had immigrated. In contrast, 20% of new psychiatrists entering the mental health workforce in Spain (Murcia) are immigrants. In Switzerland, about 50% of the psychiatrists in clinics are non-Swiss citizens. The countries reporting data on immigration are:

- Georgia, Malta, Moldova and the former Yugoslav Republic of Macedonia: none
- Hungary: less than 1%
- Luxembourg: 3%
- Spain (Extremadura): 2 %
- Spain (Murcia): 20%
- Switzerland: 50% (public sector).

Main activities initiated and developed since 2005 related to the availability of specialist mental health workers

- Albania: psychologists and social workers are placed in all mental hospitals and community-based psychiatric inpatient units.
- Bosnia and Herzegovina (Federation of Bosnia and Herzegovina): the Ministry of Health has started a situation analysis of the health workforce. The workforce has increased in size. Plans for 2006 and 2007 were to strengthen nursing competencies in mental health.
- Ireland: current staffing for mental health services is estimated at 9200. A vision for change estimates a need for about 11 000 staff members: a net increase of about 1800. A reduction in the number of nurses is envisaged, with increases in other disciplines such as consultants in psychiatry, psychology, social work, occupational therapy and other therapists.
- Luxembourg: numbers of personnel have increased substantially.
- Norway: staff members working with mental health problems have increased substantially both in specialized and in community health settings after the mental health reform. The recruitment goals of the reform have almost been achieved.

Competencies of specialist mental health workers

Undergraduate training hours on mental health

Physicians

Countries were asked to report on the undergraduate (first degree) training hours (number and proportion of the total number of undergraduate training hours) devoted to mental health (psychiatry and psychology) in educational institutions for physicians.

Information was available for 20 of 42 countries (Table 7.5). The proportion of undergraduate training hours dedicated to mental health ranges from 6% in Austria to 1.5% in Bulgaria and Moldova. The median is 3.4%.

Table 7.5. Proportion of undergraduate training hours for physicians that focus on mental health in countries

Country	Physicians' undergraduate training hours (%)
Austria	6
Poland	5–8
Portugal	5
United Kingdom (Scotland)	5
Croatia	<5
Germany	<5
Switzerland	<5
United Kingdom (England and Wales)	4.3
Uzbekistan	4.3
Spain	3.9
Turkey	3.7
Bosnia and Herzegovina	
Federation of Bosnia and Herzegovina	3.1
Republika Srpska	3.1
Estonia	3
Romania	3
The former Yugoslav Republic of Macedonia	2.7
Slovenia	2.57
Lithuania	2.45
Georgia	2.3
Albania	2
Bulgaria	1.5
Moldova	1.5

- Bulgaria: this figure (75 hours only for psychiatry) does not include practical exercises partly related to mental health in other specialties – such as medical ethics or social medicine. It is related to hours on theory only. The undergraduate programme for physicians includes 37 specialties. The postgraduate training (specialization in psychiatry) takes four years according to the state requirements for medical university training since 2005.
- Germany: the number of training hours differs in the curriculum of each medical school. To be admitted to the second part of the medical examination, candidates must prove that they have fulfilled the requirements in the fields of psychiatry and psychotherapy as well as psychosomatic medicine and psychotherapy. The individual medical schools regulate the fulfilment of these requirements (information from the German Medical Association).

Table 7.6. Number of undergraduate training hours for physicians that focus on mental health in countries

Country	Physicians' undergraduate training hours
Albania	105
Austria	225
Azerbaijan	140
Bosnia and Herzegovina	
Federation of Bosnia and Herzegovina	140
Republika Srpska	140
Bulgaria	75 only for psychiatry
Croatia	130
Estonia	280
Finland	445
Georgia	130
Germany	About 80
Hungary	300
Ireland	320 (one fifth of the final two-year medical programme)
Israel	4 hours, 3 weeks for clinical clerkship
Latvia	50 academic hours
Lithuania	144
Malta	360
Moldova	108
Norway	10 weeks of study in total during 6 years
Poland	240–376 (differs according to the curriculum of each medical university)
Portugal	265
Romania	150
Russian Federation	104 hours: 34 hours in psychology (third year) and 70 hours in psychiatry (fifth year)
Serbia	80
Slovakia	150
Slovenia	150
Spain	160
The former Yugoslav Republic of Macedonia	2 + 2 (4 training hours a week, theory and practice) in 2 semesters
Turkey	307
United Kingdom (England and Wales)	8 weeks
Uzbekistan	197

- Poland: the number of training hours differs according to the curriculum of each medical university.
- United Kingdom (Scotland): about 5% in years 3 and 4 plus special study modules available in other years.
- United Kingdom (England and Wales): for medical students there is no set number. In the 2005 survey it was very variable. The average time devoted to clinical psychiatry placements was 8 weeks (range 4–11), but 46% also said the course was integrated. Some of the newer schools have shorter placements. In the eight weeks, students were expected to attend lectures as well as gain clinical skills. Some schools include the subspecialties as part of the placement; others have that as an option. The average undergraduate course is 5 years, although teaching is usually about 30 weeks in years 1 and 2 and 42 weeks in years 3, 4 and 5, totalling about 186 weeks, of which 8 are clinical psychiatry. Many students have a few psychology lectures in earlier years, but that varies.

More countries were able to provide information on the total number of hours of undergraduate training for physicians (Table 7.6)

Nurses

The proportion of hours dedicated to mental health training is strongly correlated to the degree of nursing specialization in mental health care. It varies significantly from 66.6% in Ireland and 48.8% in United Kingdom (England and Wales) to 2% in Albania and 0% in Azerbaijan and Georgia (Tables 7.7 and 7.8).

At the top end of the figures, the percentages indicate the high level of specialization in Ireland and the United Kingdom (England and Wales) compared with the rest of the WHO European Region. At the lower end, it suggests a lack of tradition of specialist training for nurses in CIS countries, which has not yet been reversed.

- Bulgaria: training for nurses covers: 30 hours of nursing care, 30 hours of palliative care, 15 hours of problems associated with older people, 30 hours of child and adolescent medicine and medical psychology.
- France: 400 hours of obligatory theoretical psychiatry (18%) and 280 hours of obligatory clinical psychiatry.
- Germany: the structure of the training and examination regulations for the nursing profession are oriented towards individual topics and do not provide concrete indications of the number of training hours. Inpatient care in psychiatry, as a component of the practical training provided for health care and inpatient nurses, and stationary care in child and adolescent psychiatry, as a component of practical training provided for health care and children's nurses, belong to the area of differentiation. According to an estimate by the Federal Association of Nurse Directors in Psychiatric Care, the number of hours is about 60.
- Ireland: nurses' hours for programmes are based on the application by the Irish Nursing Board of EU Directive 77/453/EEC to psychiatric nurse registration and education programmes. Theoretical instruction is no less than one third of 4600 hours = 1533 hours delivered over the four years of the programme.
- Israel: 70 theoretical hours and 96 clinical hours.
- Moldova: 1.3% for psychiatry and 1.2% for psychology.
- Poland: the number of training hours differs according to the curriculum of each medical university.
- Switzerland: Training varies in the different curricula and types of schools. The Swiss Confederation's education system includes the following levels of qualification for nursing:
  - secondary level II: health practitioner EFZ – three years;
  - tertiary level B: registered nurse HF (higher vocational school) – three years (reduction possible on the basis of prior training); and
  - tertiary level A: registered nurse FH (advanced technical college) – four years (in partial transition to bachelor of nursing science (three years) and master in nursing science (two years)).

Table 7.7. Proportion of undergraduate training hours dedicated to mental health training for nurses that focus on mental health in countries

Country	Nurses' undergraduate training hours (%)
Ireland	66.6
United Kingdom (England and Wales)	48.8
France	18
Cyprus	11.5
The former Yugoslav Republic of Macedonia	11.5
Israel	11.4
Turkey	9.7
Croatia	6.5
Spain	6
Poland	5–12
Slovenia	5.3
Georgia	5
Austria	3.5
Bosnia and Herzegovina (Republika Srpska)	3.5
Estonia	3.4
Bulgaria	3.3
Lithuania	2.9
Moldova	2.5
Albania	2
Azerbaijan	0
Georgia	0

Table 7.8. Number of undergraduate training hours dedicated to mental health for nurses that focus on mental health in countries

Country	Nurses' undergraduate training hours
Albania	64
Austria	70
Azerbaijan	0
Bosnia and Herzegovina	
Federation of Bosnia and Herzegovina	105
Republika Srpska	105
Bulgaria	165
Croatia	210
Cyprus	210
Estonia	220
Finland	351
France	400 compulsory theoretical hours in psychiatry (18%) and 280 compulsory clinical hours
Georgia	0
Germany	60
Hungary	102
Ireland	1022
Israel	70 theoretical hours and 96 clinical hours
Latvia	55 academic hours
Lithuania	112
Luxembourg	15 hours in basic training
Moldova	140
Montenegro	72
Norway	About 7 weeks of study addressing psychology and educational sciences during three-year study
Poland	350–570 (differs according to the curriculum of each medical university)
Russian Federation	70 hours
Slovenia	245
Spain	135
Switzerland	
The former Yugoslav Republic of Macedonia	240
Turkey	434
United Kingdom	
England and Wales	2050
Scotland	4600

  - In addition, master of nursing science or health policy (master of public health) qualifications are offered at the university level.
  - Psychiatric issues and the promotion and maintenance of mental health are included in all curricula in a manner appropriate to the relevant level.
- The former Yugoslav Republic of Macedonia: total of 240 educational and training hours of 2070 hours for all subjects in the first six semesters.
- United Kingdom (England and Wales): as a rough estimate, mental health nurses must have 4200 hours of training, of which about 2050 hours are in mental health for the mental health branch; other branches would receive about 250–500 hours of mental health training.

Social workers

The picture for social workers is diverse, reflecting the variety of roles and responsibilities this staff group can carry, ranging from generic community workers to specialist mental health staff (Tables 7.9 and 7.10). National curricula do not always

Table 7.9. Proportion of undergraduate training hours dedicated to mental health for social workers that focus on mental health in countries

Country	Social workers' undergraduate training hours (%)
Cyprus	26
Poland	13
Slovenia	3.6 (for all; 12.7 in special department)
Germany	10
Spain (Catalonia)	10
Bosnia and Herzegovina	
Federation of Bosnia and Herzegovina	9.7
Bosnia and Herzegovina Republika Srpska	9.7
Moldova	8.6
Israel	8.5
Spain (Castilla y Léon)	7.2
Austria	5.8
Croatia	5
Turkey	4.1
The former Yugoslav Republic of Macedonia	3.3
Albania	0
Azerbaijan	0
Georgia	0

exist. This means that curricula are likely to vary considerably across training institutions within a country, which may explain the absence of data from many countries. Some of the data may therefore not be nationally representative.

Some countries without a social work tradition are now developing curricula that include a considerable mental health component.

Specialist training for psychiatrists and psychologists

Specialist training programmes in a range of areas that include the mental health of children and adolescents, the mental health of older people, forensic psychiatry, drug addiction and alcohol are available for psychiatrists in most countries (Table 7.11).

Of the 43 countries, 27 report that all these types of specialist training are available: Albania, Belgium, Bosnia and Herzegovina

Table 7.10. Number of undergraduate training hours dedicated to mental health for social workers that focus on mental health in countries

Country	Social workers' undergraduate training hours
Albania	0
Austria	10
Azerbaijan	0
Bosnia and Herzegovina	
Federation of Bosnia and Herzegovina	235 + free choice training hours devoted to mental health
Republika Srpska	235 + free choice training hours devoted to mental health
Croatia	128
Cyprus	280
Georgia	0
Germany	About 200
Hungary	300
Ireland	27 (approximate average)
Israel	11
Luxembourg	Abroad
Malta	84
Moldova	523 for psychology and 40 hours on community mental health services
Norway	18 European Credit Transfer System (ECTS) credits during three-year programme (total 180 ECTS credits) on psychology
Poland	375
Russian Federation	100 for social psychiatry (obligatory) and 75 (optional) for child psychiatry
Slovenia	120 (all or 420 in special department)
Spain	
Catalonia	185
Castilla y Léon	150
The former Yugoslav Republic of Macedonia	4 training hours per week in 2 semesters out of 8
Turkey	182
United Kingdom (England and Wales)	300–400: as an estimate 1 or 2 modules, taking into account placement learning about mental health

Table 7.11. Availability of specialist training programmes for psychiatrists in groups of countries

Topics of specialist training programmes available to psychiatrists	EU		EU15		New EU countries since 2004		Israel, Norway and Switzerland		South-eastern Europe		CIS		Total	
	No.	%	No.	%	No.	%	No.	%	No.	%	No.	%	No.	%
Child and adolescent mental health														
Yes	25	93	14	93	11	92	3	100	7	100	3	60	38	90
No	2	7	1	7	1	8	0	0	0	0	2	40	4	10
Mental health of older people														
Yes	18	67	11	73	7	58	3	100	5	71	2	40	28	67
No	9	33	4	27	5	42	0	0	2	29	3	60	14	33
Forensic psychiatry														
Yes	19	70	11	73	8	67	3	100	7	100	3	60	32	76
No	7	26	3	20	4	33	0	0	0	0	2	40	9	21
Information not available	1	4	1	7	0	0	0	0	0	0	0	0	1	2
Drug addiction														
Yes	21	78	12	80	9	75	3	100	6	86	5	100	35	83
No	6	22	3	20	3	25	0	0	1	14	0	0	7	17
Alcohol														
Yes	19	70	10	67	9	75	3	100	6	86	5	100	33	79
No	8	30	5	33	3	25	0	0	1	14	0	0	9	21

(Federation of Bosnia and Herzegovina and Republika Srpska), Cyprus, Czech Republic, Denmark, France, Germany, Hungary, Israel, Italy, Latvia, Lithuania, Montenegro, Netherlands, Norway, Poland, Portugal, Russian Federation, Serbia, Slovakia, Spain (Castilla y León, Catalonia and Murcia), Sweden, Switzerland, Turkey, United Kingdom (England, Wales and Scotland) and Uzbekistan. Only Malta and Luxembourg indicate that none of these programmes are available, but this can be attributed to the fact that psychiatrists in these countries are trained abroad (Table 7.12).

Psychologists in 13 countries (Belgium, Hungary, Ireland, Italy, Latvia, Netherlands, Norway, Russian Federation, Slovakia, Spain (Catalonia and Murcia), Switzerland, Turkey and United Kingdom (England, Wales and Scotland)) also have access to all these specialist programmes (Tables 7.13 and 7.14).

Thirteen countries (Austria, Azerbaijan, Croatia, Cyprus, Denmark, Georgia, Luxembourg, Malta, Moldova, Montenegro, Romania, Slovenia and Uzbekistan) report that none of these specialist training programmes is available for psychologists.

Since the length and content of these training programmes for psychiatrists and psychologists are not specified, these findings are not directly comparable. In the EU15 countries, Norway and Switzerland, availability means formal accreditation and registration, with a duration of at least months and sometimes years. In other countries, training can refer to short courses. For example, in Georgia an international nongovernmental organization is organizing training on children's mental health and forensic psychiatry, which is not formally accredited. In Albania, some classes are offered to psychology students, but they are not mental health education programmes. Specialist training is an area in which standardization and quality control is urgently indicated.

Continuing education

Considering the very fast pace of change in service delivery and scientific developments, continuing education is a crucial part of workforce development, comparable in importance to basic training. It could therefore be expected that this would be regulated and accredited.

Table 7.12. Training programmes available for psychiatrists in countries

Country	Training programmes available in: child and adolescent mental health	mental health of older people	forensic psychiatry	drug addiction	in alcohol
Albania	Yes	Yes	Yes	Yes	Yes
Austria	Yes	No	No	No	No
Azerbaijan	No	No	No	Yes	Yes
Belgium	Yes	Yes	Yes	Yes	Yes
Bosnia and Herzegovina					
Federation of Bosnia and Herzegovina	Yes	Yes	Yes	Yes	Yes
Republika Srpska	Yes	Yes	Yes	Yes	Yes
Bulgaria	Yes	No	Yes	Yes	Yes
Croatia	Yes	No	Yes	No	No
Cyprus	Yes	Yes	Yes	Yes	Yes
Czech Republic	Yes	Yes	Yes	Yes	Yes
Denmark	Yes	Yes	Yes	Yes	Yes
Estonia	Yes	No	No	No	No
Finland	Yes	No	Yes	No	No
France	Yes	Yes	Yes	Yes	Yes
Georgia	No	No	No	Yes	Yes
Germany	Yes	Yes	Yes	Yes	Yes
Greece	Yes	No	No	Yes	No
Hungary	Yes	Yes	Yes	Yes	Yes
Ireland	Yes	Yes	Information not available	Yes	No
Israel	Yes	Yes	Yes	Yes	Yes
Italy	Yes	Yes	Yes	Yes	Yes
Latvia	Yes	Yes	Yes	Yes	Yes
Lithuania	Yes	Yes	Yes	Yes	Yes
Luxembourg	No	No	No	No	No
Malta	No	No	No	No	No
Moldova	Yes	No	Yes	Yes	Yes
Montenegro	Yes	Yes	Yes	Yes	Yes
Netherlands	Yes	Yes	Yes	Yes	Yes
Norway	Yes	Yes	Yes	Yes	Yes
Poland	Yes	Yes	Yes	Yes	Yes
Portugal	Yes	Yes	Yes	Yes	Yes
Romania	Yes	No	No	Yes	Yes
Russian Federation	Yes	Yes	Yes	Yes	Yes
Serbia	Yes	Yes	Yes	Yes	Yes
Slovakia	Yes	Yes	Yes	Yes	Yes
Slovenia	Yes	No	No	No	No
Spain					
Castilla y León	Yes	Yes	Yes	Yes	Yes
Catalonia	Yes	Yes	Yes	Yes	Yes
Extremadura	Information not available	Information not available	Information not available	Yes	Information not available
Galicia	Yes	Yes	Information not available	Yes	Yes
Murcia	Yes	Yes	Yes	Yes	Yes
Sweden	Yes	Yes	Yes	Yes	Yes
Switzerland	Yes	Yes	Yes	Yes	Yes
The former Yugoslav Republic of Macedonia	Yes	No	Yes	Yes	Yes
Turkey	Yes	Yes	Yes	Yes	Yes
United Kingdom					
England and Wales	Yes	Yes	Yes	Yes	Yes
Scotland	Yes	Yes	Yes	Yes	Yes
Uzbekistan	Yes	Yes	Yes	Yes	Yes

Yes ■ No ■ Information not available

Table 7.13. Availability of specialist training programmes for psychologists in groups of countries

Topics of specialist training programmes available to psychologists	EU		EU15		New EU countries since 2004		Israel, Norway and Switzerland		South-eastern Europe		CIS		Total	
	No.	%	No.	%	No.	%	No.	%	No.	%	No.	%	No.	%
Child and adolescent mental health														
Yes	20	74	12	80	8	67	3	100	4	57	1	20	28	67
No	7	26	3	20	4	33	0	0	3	43	4	80	14	33
Mental health of older people														
Yes	13	48	8	53	5	42	3	100	2	29	1	20	19	45
No	12	44	7	47	5	42	0	0	4	57	4	80	20	48
Information not available	2	7	0	0	2	17	0	0	1	14	0	0	3	7
Forensic psychiatry														
Yes	12	44	6	40	6	50	2	67	2	29	1	20	17	40
No	13	48	8	53	5	42	1	33	4	57	4	80	22	52
Information not available	2	7	1	7	1	8	0	0	1	14	0	0	3	7
Drug addiction														
Yes	18	67	11	73	7	58	2	67	3	43	1	20	24	57
No	9	33	4	27	5	42	1	33	4	57	4	80	18	43
Alcohol														
Yes	17	63	10	67	7	58	2	67	4	57	1	20	24	57
No	10	37	5	33	5	42	1	33	3	43	4	80	18	43

Countries were asked to provide information about refresher training courses for different staff categories and to specify the proportion of staff with at least two days of training in the past year committed to rational use of psychotropic drugs and in psychosocial (non-biological) interventions.

The information available on the proportion of mental health staff receiving such training is limited. When data is provided, it is mostly indicative.

- Many countries indicate that, although training courses do take place, the number of staff attending them is not available, since it is not recorded.
- A broad mix of activities accounts for refresher training and continuing education: from presentation of new drugs organized by pharmaceutical companies to attendance at conferences or training seminars on specific topics.
- Although nurses in most countries have a duty to undertake a certain number of training hours every year, they do not have to be in mental health – they could be in violence management or in infectious diseases.
- Very few countries report regulation of continuing medical education, linked to the right to practise (Germany, the Netherlands, Switzerland).

We asked about the number of psychiatrists with at least two days of training in the last year in the rational use of psychotropic drugs and in psychosocial (non-biological) interventions

The following countries made comments.

- Albania: there is no system of continuing education for either psychiatrists or nurses.
- Austria: information is not available. Participation in refreshers is up to doctors. Continuing medical education is compulsory for all licensed doctors, but there are no penalties when doctors do not renew their continuing medical education diplomas. A number of continuing medical education interventions are offered in Austria's continuing medical education calendar.
- Azerbaijan: such training courses are not available.

Table 7.14. Training programmes available for psychologists in countries

Country	Training programmes available in: child and adolescent mental health	mental health of older people	forensic psychiatry	drug addiction	alcohol
Albania	No	No	Yes	No	Yes
Austria	No	No	No	No	No
Azerbaijan	No	No	No	No	No
Belgium	Yes	Yes	Yes	Yes	Yes
Bosnia and Herzegovina					
Federation of Bosnia and Herzegovina	Yes	Yes	No	Yes	Yes
Republika Srpska	Yes	Yes	No	Yes	Yes
Bulgaria	Yes	Information not available	Yes	Yes	Yes
Croatia	No	No	No	No	No
Cyprus	No	No	No	No	No
Czech Republic	Yes	Information not available	Yes	Yes	Yes
Denmark	No	No	No	No	No
Estonia	Yes	No	No	No	No
Finland	Yes	No	No	No	No
France	Yes	No	No	Yes	Yes
Georgia	No	No	No	No	No
Germany	Yes	No	No	Yes	Yes
Greece	Yes	No	No	Yes	No
Hungary	Yes	Yes	Yes	Yes	Yes
Ireland	Yes	Yes	Yes	Yes	Yes
Israel	Yes	Yes	No	No	No
Italy	Yes	Yes	Yes	Yes	Yes
Latvia	Yes	Yes	Yes	Yes	Yes
Lithuania	Yes	Yes	Information not available	Yes	Yes
Luxembourg	No	No	No	No	No
Malta	No	No	No	No	No
Moldova	No	No	No	No	No
Montenegro	No	No	No	No	No
Netherlands	Yes	Yes	Yes	Yes	Yes
Norway	Yes	Yes	Yes	Yes	Yes
Poland	Yes	Yes	Yes	Yes	Yes
Portugal	Yes	Yes	No	Yes	Yes
Romania	No	No	No	No	No
Russian Federation	Yes	Yes	Yes	Yes	Yes
Serbia	Yes	Information not available	Information not available	Yes	Yes
Slovakia	Yes	Yes	Yes	Yes	Yes
Slovenia	No	No	No	No	No
Spain					
Castilla y León	Yes	Yes	Information not available	Yes	Information not available
Catalonia	Yes	Yes	Yes	Yes	Yes
Extremadura	Information not available	Information not available	Information not available	Information not available	Information not available
Galicia	Yes	Yes	Information not available	Yes	Yes
Murcia	Yes	Yes	Yes	Yes	Yes
Sweden	Yes	Yes	Information not available	Yes	Yes
Switzerland	Yes	Yes	Yes	Yes	Yes
The former Yugoslav Republic of Macedonia	Yes	No	No	No	No
Turkey	Yes	Yes	Yes	Yes	Yes
United Kingdom					
England and Wales	Yes	Yes	Yes	Yes	Yes
Scotland	Yes	Yes	Yes	Yes	Yes
Uzbekistan	No	No	No	No	No

Yes No Information not available

- Bulgaria: there is not sufficient information, although these activities take place. Various institutions or interested groups such as professional organizations, pharmaceutical companies etc. organize refresher training courses. It is a part of continuing medical education, which is organized based on credit points that have to be collected during the year. The Bulgarian Medical Association issues the credits, being responsible for the continuing medical education according to the Law on Professional Organizations. The Bulgarian Medical Association does not aggregate the information and keeps it as personal registries maintained by each regional professional organization.
- Croatia: courses are available, but no data on the number of participants.
- Denmark: there are courses on both subjects but the numbers are not known.
- France: there is continuing medical education in these fields for all the professionals, but this cannot be quantified.
- Israel: there are no formal requirements for mental health workers regarding refresher training. There are local education programmes organized by unit management, sickness funds, etc.
- Italy: precise data are only available at level of mental health departments.
- Luxembourg: probably more than 50% for both, but no official data are available.
- Malta: psychiatrists participate in conferences sponsored by pharmaceutical companies, but no record and no formal structure.
- Netherlands: a registry for meeting continuing medical education standards is maintained for individual psychiatrists, essential for the right to practice.
- Poland: each year, a number of refresher courses for psychiatrists are organized as well as conferences on current problems of treatment and care, but the proportion of staff participating is not available. Physicians are obliged to adhere to continuing education.
- Russian Federation: every fifth year, every psychiatrist should take a comprehensive certification course on psychiatry (90–190 hours). The programme of such mandatory courses includes these issues. Besides that, refresher courses are available once every 1–5 years (depending on the region).
- Serbia – continuing medical education courses for psychiatrists are organized regularly, at least once a month across the country.
- Switzerland: psychiatrists are required to undertake further training annually.
- The former Yugoslav Republic of Macedonia: there is occasional training but not on a regular basis and not on an institutionalized basis.
- United Kingdom (England and Wales): the Royal College of Psychiatrists registers members for Continuing Professional Development, but the content of this is the choice of the individual.

We asked about the number of nurses with at least two days of training in the last year in the rational use of psychotropic drugs and in psychosocial (non-biological) interventions.

The following countries made comments.

- Croatia: courses available but no data on the number of participants.
- France: there is continuing education in these fields for all the professionals, but this cannot be quantified.
- Israel: there are no formal requirements for mental health workers regarding refresher training. There are local educational programmes organized by unit management, trade unions, sickness funds, etc.
- Netherlands: courses are available, but the details are not available.
- Poland: each year, a number of refresher courses for nurses working in mental health are organized but the proportion of staff participating is not available.
- Russian Federation: training undertaken, but exact data are not available.
- Switzerland: unlike basic training, retraining and professional development training for nurses is not regulated (not obligatory). There are opportunities for retraining and professional development training in psychiatry and mental health for all the levels of qualification, and these are used. These options are developed

Table 7.15. Availability of training programmes for personnel that are organized and conducted in partnership with service users, former service users and carers in groups of countries

Training programmes available	EU		EU15		New EU countries since 2004		Israel, Norway and Switzerland		South-eastern Europe		CIS		Total	
	No.	%	No.	%	No.	%	No.	%	No.	%	No.	%	No.	%
Yes	8	30	7	47	1	8	2	67	3	43	1	20	14	33
No	13	48	5	33	8	67	1	33	3	43	4	80	21	50
Information not available	6	22	3	20	3	25	0	0	1	14	0	0	7	17

and provided by the relevant training institutions (vocational training centers, higher vocational schools, advanced technical colleges), by regional professional development training centers and by the Swiss Nurses' Association. The focus and intensity of such professional development can be directed by cantonal or regional psychiatric planning and the needs of the various psychiatric or psychosocial care institutions.

- United Kingdom (Scotland): to maintain registration, all qualified mental health nurses must undertake at least 35 hours of training in the previous three years.

Training programmes for staff that are organized and conducted in partnership with service users, former service users and carers

In the Mental Health Declaration for Europe, Member States identify as one of the five priorities for the WHO European Region "recognizing the experience and knowledge of service users and carers as an important basis for planning and developing mental health services".

Of the 43 countries, 15 (35%) report that some training programmes for staff members are organized and conducted in partnership with service users and carers (Table 7.13). The information collected does not establish whether this is common practice in any of these countries and whether they are organized in the framework of mainstream training for mental health staff or in the context of pilot initiatives coordinated by nongovernmental organizations.

Main activities initiated and developed since 2005 related to education and training and the development of competencies

Development of training curricula

- Update of training curricula in public health and psychiatry (Bosnia and Herzegovina (Federation of Bosnia and Herzegovina and Republika Srpska).
- Introduction of community mental health module (Bosnia and Herzegovina (Federation of Bosnia and Herzegovina and Republika Srpska) and the former Yugoslav Republic of Macedonia)
- In Ireland, the Health Service Executive has taken steps to expand the availability of multidisciplinary team members, such as stabilizing and rationalizing clinical psychology training with the National University of Ireland, Trinity College Dublin, University of Limerick and National University of Ireland, Galway.
- In Romania, a new education programme for the mental health of children and adolescents has been available since 2007 for health professionals with three years of education from different fields.
- In Spain (Extremadura), establishment of a master degree in social medicine (Atención Sociosanitaria).
- In the United Kingdom (Scotland), many frameworks on capability, competencies and educational resources have been developed for mental health nursing.
- In Uzbekistan, programmes of basic and postgraduate education of physicians and other health care staff, including psychiatrists and psychotherapists, were reviewed in 2007.

Organizing training

- Albania: Training of staff working in primary health care and refresher training for mental health workers.
- Serbia: the Institute of Mental Health regularly organizes the education and training of mental health professionals and GPs.
- Georgia:
  - Training of mental health nurses - a pilot initiative sponsored by Global Initiative on Psychiatry, an international nongovernmental organization focusing on protecting the human rights of users in mental health services.
  - Implementing a three-year programme for training in the mental health of children and forensic psychiatry for psychiatrists and psychologists (developed by Global Initiative in Psychiatry and sponsored by Cordaid, an international development foundation).
  - A new education programme for the mental health of children and adolescents has been available since 2007 for health professionals with three years of education from different fields (sponsored by Norway).
- Luxembourg: continuing education programmes extended.
- Poland: Training programmes in the mental health of older people for psychiatrists and psychologists.
- Spain (Catalonia): increase in the number of training places.
- Croatia: establishment of the Centre for Education on Psychosocial Rehabilitation.
- Ireland: the Health Service Executive and Mental Health Commission are funding a research project with the University of Limerick on the current reality of multidisciplinary team functioning in Ireland.
- United Kingdom (England): in recent years, a national programme of work has been undertaken to help support the mental health workforce across health and social care. This has taken numerous forms, but primarily the focus has been on developing New Ways of Working (the NWW programme, http://newwaysofworking.org.uk), where responsibility is distributed among members of the mental health team with a move to ensure that the most advanced skills are deployed to deal with the most complex cases and the provision of supervision or support to the rest of the team; the introduction of new roles to help meet specific needs of service users and carers and to help expand the workforce; the introduction of the Creating Capable Teams Approach (CCTA) that helps mental health teams focus on the needs of service users and carers and of the capabilities that exist within the team; and the learning and development needs of staff using the foundation of the Ten Essential Shared Capabilities framework that all staff are expected to adopt as part of their everyday practice supported by learning materials on the Ten Essential Shared Capabilities; the recovery approach; social inclusion; and race equality and cultural capability.

Discussion

The most striking observations in this chapter are the variation in staff numbers, differences in education and the lack of reliable information available from countries in many areas.

Surprisingly, at a time of reform and rapid change in the numbers, composition and competencies of the workforce, in combination with ubiquitous concern about recruiting adequate numbers of staff members, fewer than half the countries in this survey have produced a mental health workforce strategy. The components of such strategies may be incorporated into overall mental health strategies, presented in an earlier chapter, or generic workforce strategies not enquired about in this survey, but this still would leave concern about some of the specific mental health workforce issues that need to be addressed in some detail during the next few years.

Despite the similarities in strategic direction across countries, as symbolized by the endorsement of the Mental Health Declaration for Europe, it is striking how the numbers in each staff group vary across the WHO European Region, even between countries with comparable wealth and development of mental health services. The rates of psychiatrists turn out to be quite variable, despite their professional registration in all countries, which should guarantee some reliability. Despite agreement on definitions, the registration process in countries may have included or excluded different categories of psychiatrists, such as inactive or retired psychiatrists or those employed outside the public sector. Nevertheless, there are still some major differences in numbers that cannot be explained by misclassification, reflecting variation in the role of psychiatrists, health system differences including reimbursement practices, salaries and workforce planning such as number of training places.

All countries take the training of psychiatrists seriously, although the time invested in undergraduate training varies considerably, which is likely to reflect the competencies of GPs and other physicians. The duration of psychiatric specialization, which was not included in this survey, is more comparable, particularly across the EU, and organizations such as the European Union of Medical Specialists (EUMS) are active in proposing international curricula and quality control. Many non-EU countries offer considerably shorter and very different models of psychiatric training.

Subspecialization for psychiatrists and psychologists shows an optimistic picture of wide availability. These data and similar data need to be interpreted very carefully, since the recognition of subspecialization stands for a long period of training in some countries, typically 1–3 years, followed by registration as a subspecialist. Others rely on brief courses, non-accredited, offered by independent agencies. Attaining some form of standardization is a great challenge.

Sometimes answers suggest superficial similarities. The survey asked a question about training for nurses and physicians provided in community settings, which has been omitted since the large majority of countries answered affirmatively. It proved impossible to distinguish between countries that offered training in community teams versus polyclinics or general hospitals, all interpreted variably as standing for community services. At this stage of highly differentiated services and reforms, one country's community care service is another country's institution.

Several of the points made for psychiatrists can be made more strongly for nurses. Predictably, the numbers vary. However, two issues stand out for nursing education that have implications for the quality of care. First, it is surprising how many countries cannot provide data about numbers. Second, the training and levels of education differ vastly, raising questions about competencies in some countries. Some countries train mental health nurses to a high degree of specialization, whereas others hardly include any time on this subject in the nursing curriculum. This raises concerns for local practice as well as workforce migration.

As this report demonstrates, the situation for other staff groups is even more ambiguous, either due to their generic roles, not limited to mental health, or because these groups have only recently been established and do not yet exist in practical terms in some countries. The variation in the numbers of psychologists is an example of this. Establishing training places, curricula and positions in mental health care for a sufficient number of psychologists, social workers and occupational therapists is clearly an urgent priority.

Apart from international variation, medical schools and other training institutions for psychiatrists and other staff groups within countries also vary significantly, creating graduates with a unique set of attitudes and skills. Whether this is desirable or not can be debated, but unquestionably it could lead to unpredictable results unless competencies are standardized and ascertained.

At a time of vast change in service delivery and knowledge, continuing education is important. No one would like to be operated on by a surgeon educated 25 years ago who has had no more recent updated training. The picture drawn by the information gathered on continuing education in this survey is not reassuring. Continuing education seems to be taking place, but there is little control over content or providers, with a strong reliance on informal self-regulation. Where more formal processes have been put in place, the emphasis seems to be on the process rather than the outcome.

A subject that is raising much international concern is migration of the workforce. It is therefore surprising that few countries could provide us with information. The data available may underrepresent the scale of the challenge.

In summary, this chapter gives an impression of variation in numbers and competencies across the WHO European Region. Much of this variation is unintentional, based on tradition and status quo. Much information is unavailable. This may become important at a time of reform when new dynamics need to be planned and delivered. The lack of information in some areas may also be of concern when transnational challenges need to be resolved. Many challenges remain in this field.

"There is an absence of regulation of continuing education despite the differences in structure and roles. Continuing education seems to be open to any supplier willing to invest"

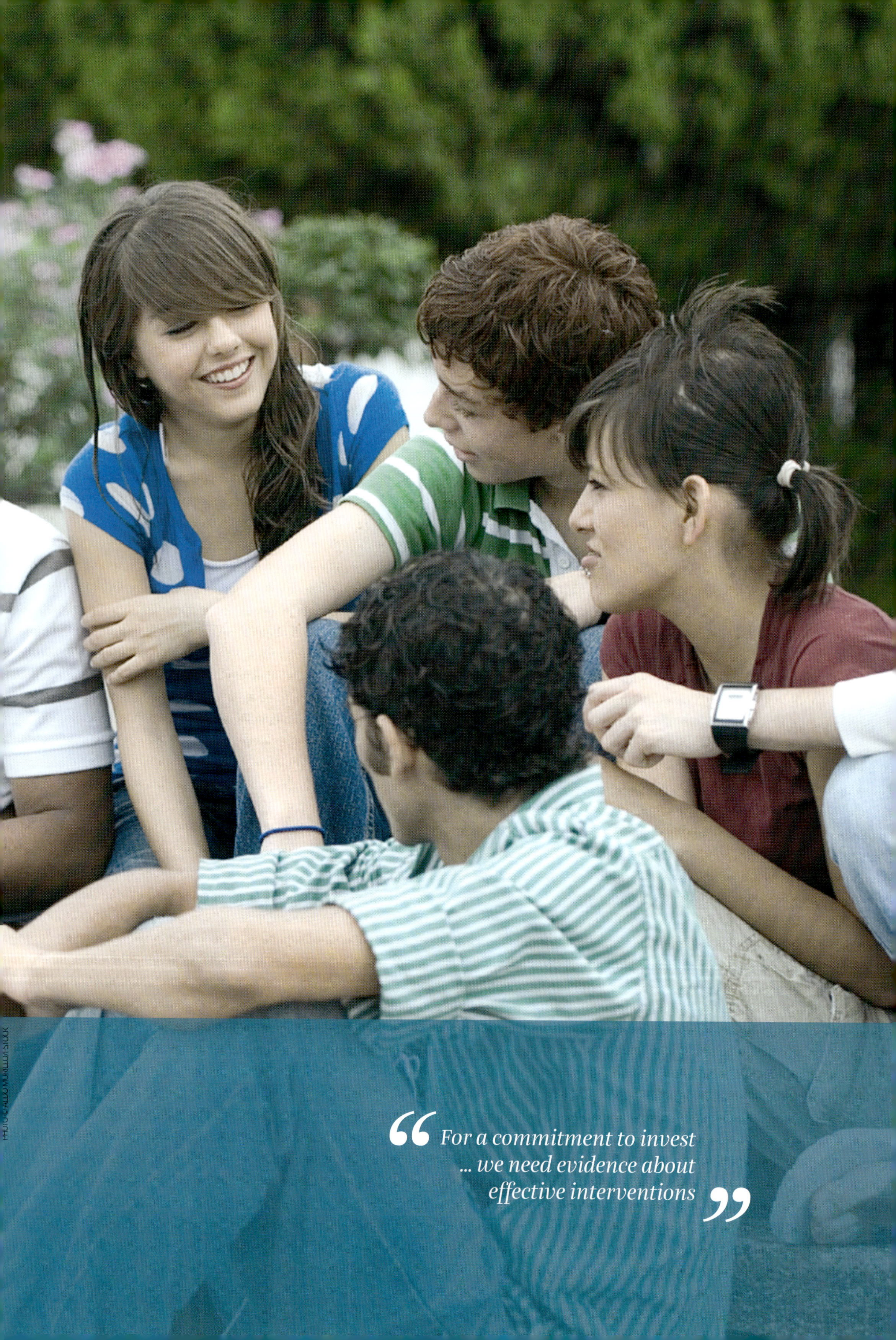

PHOTO © ALDO MURILLO/ISTOCK

8. Funding of mental health services

Reforming mental health care requires the scrutiny of costs and spending on mental health services. Traditionally, a very large proportion of the budget had been allocated to operating mental hospitals, mostly as a block grant, based on historical spending rather than need. Gradually, as a consequence of the closure of hospital beds and the development of community-based forms of care, money was shifted to community services, with declining proportions spend on mental hospital care. Simplistically, a declining proportion of the mental health budget allocated to hospital care may indicate reform.

This shift from a monolithic provision to diverse services from a range of providers, typically combining state, local and independent agencies, meant that public authorities had to make choices about budget allocation. The needs-based approach of community services resulted in pressure to increase capacity, diversity and quality, with implications for the budget. A first step was transparency about spending.

A challenge in analysing mental health budgets is that only a proportion of the mental health money comes from the health budget, and the move towards community-based services increases the need for decentralized spending. For example, local government and government departments responsible for social care are often responsible for accommodation and day care. Local spending on welfare and social care can also be increased by local taxes. These figures are very hard to identify, since they are rarely ring-fenced, and this hides the real public cost of mental health care.

This survey focused on the health budgets and expenditure and attempted to identify spending on a variety of services to determine the diversification of mental health care.

Mental health budget or expenditure as a proportion of the total health budget or expenditure

This survey asked about the mental health budget or expenditure as a proportion of the total public health budget or expenditure. Although budget and expenditure are technically different, not all countries had a budget allocated for mental health, and expenditure can be assumed to be a close approximation. The years are the latest available, mostly 2004–2006.

Some countries with a decentralized health care system and countries with a federal structure could not provide this information. In these countries, budgets are established at the local or regional level, and data on these are not always collected nationally. Some countries had information for some particular regions (for example, Bosnia and Herzegovina (Federation of Bosnia and Herzegovina) informed about the Tuzla Region). If proxies were available, these are specified in the comments column (Table 8.1, Fig. 8.1).

Countries had great difficulty in being precise about numerators and denominators. Although the requested denominator was the total health budget, some countries could only provide specialist or secondary care budgets. If countries specified in the comment column that mental health in primary care is not included in the numerator, the overall primary care budget may have been omitted from the denominator, as is the case in England and Wales.

The comment on the numerator did not always specify what services are included and excluded, especially if expenditure was not a central responsibility. Although information on some components of the budget or expenditure may be mostly available (such as for inpatient services), other components of the mental health budget were harder to find. Particularly difficult to identify were:

- mental health services provided in primary care, which represent a significant part of overall mental health care in some countries;
- reimbursement of drugs;
- private psychiatric practices contracted by health insurance;
- some outpatient services;
- mental care in nursing homes;
- expenditure on mental health promotion programmes or mental disorder prevention programmes;

Table 8.1. Mental health budget or expenditure as a percentage of the total health budget or expenditure in countries

Country	Share of the total health budget or expenditure (%)	Specification: budget or expenditure	Comments
Albania	3.0	Expenditure	The 3% refers to the percentage of the expenditure from Ministry of Health sources. Therefore, the expenditure on drugs (which accounts for another 3%) is not included here. The expenditure for drugs comes from the Health Insurance Fund budget, deriving directly from the Ministry of Finance.
Austria	Information not available		
Azerbaijan	3	Budget	
Belgium	Information not available		
Bosnia and Herzegovina			
Federation of Bosnia and Herzegovina	4.7	Expenditure	Total health expenditure was 8.8% of gross domestic product. The available data is for one region (Tuzla, with 446 830 insured inhabitants).
Republika Srpska	5.1 (of secondary health care budget); 1.85 of (primary health care budget)	Budget	
Bulgaria	2	Expenditure	Inpatient mental health care is 0.65% of total expenditure. This does not include outpatient care, psychotropic drugs or out-of-pocket payments. A rough estimate is about 2%.
Croatia	Information not available		
Cyprus	8.2	Budget	
Czech Republic	3.6	Expenditure	
Denmark	7.5	Expenditure	
Estonia	4.2	Expenditure	
Finland	Information not available		Due to the decentralized health care system, there is no national health expenditure budget. Each municipality has its own budget, and mental health budgets cannot be separated from the total health budgets.
France	11.5		The proportion represented by the expenditure budget of the institutions practising in psychiatry in all public and private health institutions is 11.5%. This does not include general practitioners, privately practising psychiatrists or reimbursement of drugs.
Georgia	4.0	Budget	
Germany	10.3	Expenditure	
Greece	Information not available		
Hungary	5.1	Expenditure and reimbursement	
Ireland	7.7	Budget	
Israel	6.1	Budget	
Italy	5.0	Budget	The target agreed (but only achieved by few regions) is to achieve 5% of the total health budget. At the national level, data are collected on expenditure, with reference to three major areas: ambulatory and home care, semi-residential care and residential care.

Country	Share of the total health budget or expenditure (%)	Specification: budget or expenditure	Comments
Latvia	6.0	Budget	
Lithuania	9.0	Expenditure	For mental health and nervous system health. In the absence of comprehensive and accurate data, a share of public expenditure for mental health could be estimated as 9% of the total.
Luxembourg	Information not available		
Malta	6.0	Budget	Refers to recurrent expenditure only.
Moldova	4	Budget	
Montenegro	Information not available		
Netherlands	8.0	Budget	
Norway	Information not available		
Poland	3.5	Expenditure	This data does not cover reimbursement of psychotropic medicines purchased in pharmacies
Portugal	3.0	Expenditure	
Romania	3.0	Budget	This excludes special funds allocated through the National Programme for Mental Health for establishing community-based mental health services and improving hospital infrastructure.
Russian Federation	5.0	Expenditure	Of the total health expenditure, expenditure for psychiatry is about 5%. This figure does not include older people's homes.
Serbia	Information not available		
Slovakia	7.1		
Slovenia	Information not available		
Spain			
Catalonia	10.5	Expenditure	
Extremadura	5.9	Budget	
Murcia	3.1	Expenditure	
Castilla y Léon	Information not available		
Galicia	Information not available		
Sweden	10.0	Expenditure	
Switzerland	9.1	Expenditure	Mental health expenditure refers to the sum of expenditure on inpatient and outpatient care and psychotropic drugs. The figure does not include mental care in nursing homes or health promotion and mental disorder prevention programmes (due to lacking data).
The former Yugoslav Republic of Macedonia	Information not available		
Turkey	Information not available		There is no separate budget for mental health expenditure. There is an overall health expenditure budget, and mental health expenditure is funded from this budget.
United Kingdom			
England and Wales	13.8	Expenditure	Proportion of the specialist budget. This figure does not include primary care or local authority spending.
Scotland	9.5	Budget	This excludes the budget for primary care and expenditure from local authorities.
Uzbekistan	2.2	Budget	From 0.76% in Jizzakh region to 4.39% in Tashkent city.

Fig. 8.1. Mental health budget or expenditure as a proportion of the total health budget or expenditure in countries

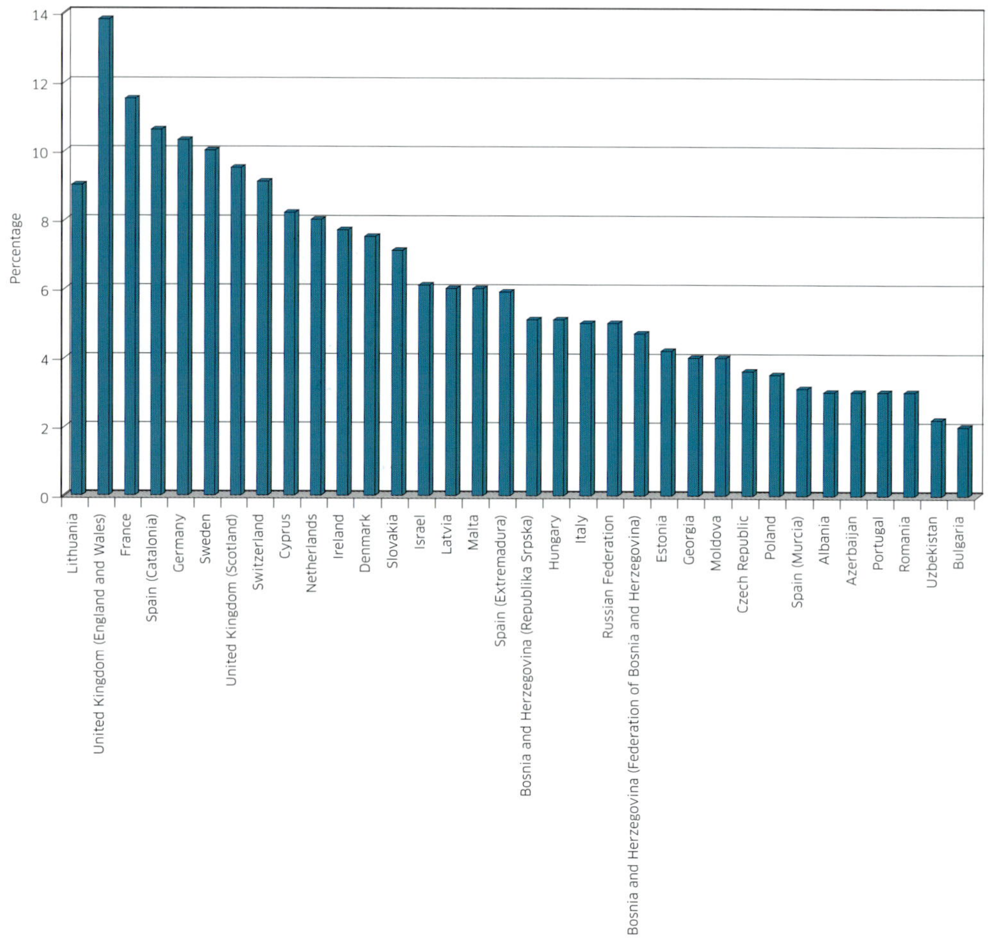

- expenditure from local authorities; and
- out-of-pocket expenditure (formal or informal).

The mental health budget figures include such components inconsistently across countries. Any cross-country comparisons should therefore be made with caution. The budget probably approximates central mental health expenditure but often underestimates total expenditure on mental health. The more advanced the community-based care and primary care mental health services and the more decentralized the funding of mental health services, the higher the additional expenditure is likely to be.

Allocation of the national mental health budget or expenditure (or aggregated regional or local budgets)

The distribution of the budget or expenditure would be more informative about investment in services than overall budget allocation.

Most countries have had difficulty in providing funding allocation for different components. This survey asked for a breakdown of the budget in the latest year available by:

- psychiatric beds in general hospitals
- mental hospitals
- community-based services (excluding beds)
- mental health care in primary care services

Table 8.2. Allocation of mental health expenditure for all psychiatric beds in all settings and those in district general hospitals in countries

Country	Mental health expenditure used for psychiatric beds (%)	
	All settings	District general hospitals
Albania	97	Information not available
Portugal	89	44.5
Azerbaijan	85	0
Moldova	85	0
Latvia	80	Information not available
Bosnia and Herzegovina (Republika Srpska)	80	32.6
Poland	78.1	Information not available
Georgia	76	0
Sweden	70	70
Bosnia and Herzegovina (Federation of Bosnia and Herzegovina)	68.7	Information not available
Malta	67	17
Czech Republic	63	10
United Kingdom (Scotland)	62.5	7.1
Switzerland	59	8.4
Spain (Extremadura)	43	Information not available
Cyprus	43	7.5
Bulgaria	38	8.2
Lithuania	38	Information not available
Germany	32	Information not available
Spain (Catalonia)	30.4	9.8
Estonia	28	Information not available
United Kingdom (England and Wales)	26	Information not available

- residential beds or nursing homes
- mental health promotion programmes
- mental disorder prevention programmes
- psychotropic drugs
- others.

The responses countries provided reflected the differences in funding mechanisms across Europe and the specificity of information.

In some countries different services are funded from the same pot – the amounts cannot be disaggregated. In other countries, information on some service components is not available, either because other funders (such as for social care institutions) are responsible or (if within the health sector) because complicated analysis would be required – which is beyond the capacity of this project.

The service component for which information is most frequently available is mental hospital beds. Twenty-two countries provided information on the proportion of the mental health budget allocated to all mental hospitals and psychiatric beds in district general hospitals (Table 8.2).

Some countries appear to allocate a very high proportion of expenditure to beds in hospitals. In many cases, such as Albania, this is due to great mental hospital expenditure. In some instances this can be explained by spending on district general hospitals. Table 8.2 shows the proportion of spending on district general hospitals for the 13 countries that provided the disaggregated data, showing mostly high expenditure on mental hospitals. However, several countries with few mental hospitals and high expenditure on district general hospitals, such as Italy and England, are not included. The 89% of expenditure by Portugal is almost equally split between mental hospitals and district general hospitals. The 70% identified by Sweden is all spent on district general hospitals. Presumably the district general hospital budgets in both countries also include some community services funded from the district general hospital budget, which could not be identified separately.

Some budget calculations can result in misleading percentages. The low percentage of hospital expenditure in Bulgaria may be due to medication being excluded from hospital expenditure, since it is considered a separate budget line.

Very few countries provided meaningful information on the remaining components. Ten countries specified spending on community-based services excluding beds, which ranged from 30% in Sweden to 0% in Georgia and Moldova. The median was 9%. However, the interpretation of the coverage of this funding, which did not include contributions from other sources such as local governments, varies to such an extent that this data cannot meaningfully be interpreted.

Four countries provided the proportion of spending on residential beds or nursing homes: the Czech Republic 2.0% (includes homes for psychiatric patients and community residential care, partly social funds of local authorities), Germany: 33.0% and United Kingdom (England and Wales): 14.0% (National Health Service 52%, local authorities 48%). Malta spent 0%, reflecting its high spending on mental hospitals.

Information on mental health promotion and mental disorder prevention programmes was not available for 88% (37 of 42) of the participating countries. For the few countries that provided these data, the combined percentages of budget allocated to mental health promotion and mental disorder prevention programmes were typically about or below 1%.

Information on expenditure on psychotropic drugs was not available for 81% of the countries (34 of 42). The percentages of the total mental health budget ranged from 3% in Germany, 7% in Moldova and 12.4% in Switzerland to 20% in Estonia, 23% in the Czech Republic and 37% in Lithuania. The variation is likely to be due to a combination of the absolute level of the budget and the ability to absorb the relatively high cost of medication (Germany), supply restrictions and co-payments (Moldova) and high levels of prescribing of antidepressants (Lithuania).

Free access (at least 80% covered) to psychotropic medication and psychotherapy

The survey asked about financial access to psychotropic medication and psychotherapy, in particular whether they are free of charge at the point of access in mental hospitals, in community services and in primary care.

Medication

All the countries reported that the public sector pays at least 80% of the cost of psychotropic medication in mental hospitals. Most countries (33 of 42, 79%) also report that at least 80% of the cost of medication is covered in community services and 34 of 42 countries (81%) in primary care (Table 8.3). Supply may nevertheless be a problem in some of the less affluent countries, where hospitals and pharmacies may not be able to offer the medication to which people are entitled. The following are a few examples.

Hospital settings

- Azerbaijan: according to legislation and rules, psychotropic medication is free of charge in hospitals. However, hospitals are poorly stocked with medication, and people therefore often have to buy medication in pharmacies.
- Bulgaria: in inpatient care, drug therapy is included in the overall treatment plan. The allocation between drug reimbursement and other therapeutic interventions, especially psychosocial rehabilitation, heavily favours drugs – more than 60% of the total expenditure is on drugs.
- Lithuania: different tariffs. People with schizophrenia do not pay for medicine. People with organic psychoses pay 50% of the cost.

Community services

- Austria: a co-payment is necessary.
- Bulgaria: in outpatient care, the National Health Insurance Fund covers the cost of the psychotropic drugs up to 100% for severe mental disorders prescribed by specialists. General practitioners can also prescribe them free of charge when referred by specialists.

Table 8.3. Psychotropic medication free of charge (at least 80% covered by public funds) in community services and primary care in groups of countries

Psychotropic medication free of charge	EU		EU15		New EU countries since 2004		Israel, Norway and Switzerland		South-eastern Europe		CIS		Total	
	No.	%	No.	%	No.	%	No.	%	No.	%	No.	%	No.	%
Community services														
Yes	21	78	14	93	7	58	2	67	7	100	3	60	33	79
No	3	11	1	7	2	17	0	0	0	0	1	20	4	10
Not applicable	0	0	0	0	0	0	0	0	0	0	1	20	1	2
Information not available	3	11	0	0	3	25	1	33	0	0	0	0	4	10
Primary care														
Yes	23	85	13	87	10	83	2	67	7	100	2	40	34	81
No	3	11	2	13	1	8	0	0	0	0	3	60	6	14
Information not available	1	4	0	0	1	8	1	33	0	0	0	0	2	5

- The former Yugoslav Republic of Macedonia: the situation in the community mental health services is almost the same as in the hospital setting as described above.
- Lithuania: in outpatient care, according to the lists approved by Ministry of Health, medicines are reimbursed 100%, 90%, 80% or 50%. For people with schizophrenia and schizoaffective disorders, all antipsychotic drugs (including all new neuroleptics) are covered 100%, severe depressive or bipolar disorders 80% and organic psychoses 50%. The person who needs the medicine must pay the difference. If the medicine is not on the list of reimbursable medicine, the person who needs the medicine pays for it.
- Poland: in hospitals and intermediate care facilities such as day treatment and care units, funded by public sources, all medicines are free of charge.
- Russian Federation: in the state health care system (not in the private sector).

Primary care

- Bosnia and Herzegovina – Federation of Bosnia and Herzegovina: drugs on the list approved by the Ministry of Health are reimbursed, but this varies from region to region.
- Denmark: only antidepressant and antipsychotic medicines are eligible for general reimbursement. General reimbursement means that people automatically get reimbursement for medicine according to the different reimbursement rates determined for each product (such as 50%, 75% or 85% reimbursement) at a pharmacy. People with chronic diseases, children and older people can get up to 100% reimbursement.
- Finland: the Social Insurance Institution of Finland reimburses people for part of the cost of necessary medication prescribed by a doctor.
- Hungary: GPs can prescribe psychotropic medication with a higher reimbursement rate for a limited time period if a board-certified psychiatrist will initiate it and evaluates it periodically.
- Italy: only benzodiazepines are not free of charge.
- Poland: in primary care, the situation varies from free of charge up to full price and depends on the type of medicine and the extent to which the disease is chronic. Medicines on the list approved by the Ministry of Health are reimbursed.

Psychotherapy

Psychotherapy can be accessed in hospitals with public funds paying at least 80% of the cost in 34 of 42 countries (81%) (Table 8.4). Fewer countries (27 of 42, 64%) report this in community services. This includes 12 of the 15 (80%) EU15 countries and 5 of the 12 (42%) countries that joined the EU after 2004. Fewer countries (20 of 42, 48%) indicate that psychotherapy is free of charge in primary care.

Table 8.4. Psychotherapy free of charge (at least 80% covered by public funds) in hospitals, community services and primary care in groups of countries

Psychotherapy free of charge	EU		EU15		New EU countries since 2004		Israel, Norway and Switzerland		South-eastern Europe		CIS		Total	
	No.	%	No.	%	No.	%	No.	%	No.	%	No.	%	No.	%
Hospitals														
Yes	23	85	14	93	9	75	2	67	6	86	3	60	34	81
No	4	15	1	7	3	25	0	0	1	14	2	40	7	17
Information not available	0	0	0	0	0	0	1	33	0	0	0	0	1	2
Community services														
Yes	17	63	12	80	5	42	2	67	6	86	2	40	27	64
No	8	30	3	20	5	42	0	0	1	14	3	60	12	29
Information not available	2	7	0	0	2	17	1	33	0	0	0	0	3	7
Primary care														
Yes	11	41	7	47	4	33	2	67	5	71	2	40	20	48
No	14	52	7	47	7	58	0	0	2	29	3	60	19	45
Information not available	2	7	1	7	1	8	1	33	0	0	0	0	3	7

In hospital

- Bulgaria: the National Health Insurance Fund does not pay for psychotherapy. In the hospital, psychotherapy is part of the rehabilitation activities before discharge.
- Hungary: extremely limited availability.
- Italy: this only refers to treatment in acute crisis settings directed by the community-based department.
- Portugal: psychotherapy is covered at least 80% by public funds but is not available at all hospitals.
- United Kingdom (England and Wales): psychotherapy is free of charge in the National Health Service, fee-for-service in the private sector and low and variable fees in various charitable clinics.

Community services

- Austria: available in some services (no general rules).
- Belgium: there is discrimination between psychiatrist psychotherapists (covered) and non-psychiatrist psychotherapists (not covered).
- Denmark: it is free of charge from GPs and psychiatrists.
- Finland: included in public services but availability is limited.
- Hungary: extremely limited availability.
- Italy: does not apply in Italy. Outside the public specialist system, people have to pay for private psychotherapy.
- Lithuania: after a psychiatrist prescribes psychotherapy, the Health Insurance Fund covers up to 24 psychotherapy sessions per year for one person according to tariffs certified by the Ministry of Health. Very few mental health centres provide psychotherapy services; they are mostly provided privately.
- Luxembourg: if provided by a psychiatrist and not if provided by a psychologist.
- Netherlands: self-employed psychotherapists in the community. Primary care psychologists will become available.
- Portugal: psychotherapy is covered at least 80% by public funds but is not available at all in community services.
- Switzerland: psychotherapy that is anticipated to last longer than 10 sessions must be reported after the sixth session to the medical examiner of the relevant insurer. This report serves simultaneously as an application for approval of the assumption of costs for 30 further sessions initially. Thereafter, a more complete report to the medical examiner and a further application for approval of the assumption of costs is required. For really long-term

therapy, a report is required at least annually.
- United Kingdom (England and Wales): free of charge where available; investment in the Improving Access to Psychological Therapies (IAPT) programme is currently addressing high levels of underprovision.
- Uzbekistan: provision with psychotherapists is extremely insufficient, and there are none in communities.

Allocation of the local or regional budget for mental health based on a formula taking into account the relative needs of the population

Several countries note that the budget allocation is based on a needs assessment of the target population, although little specification is offered, and most do not use formulas (Table 8.5).

In Croatia, there is no actual formula, and local authorities estimate specific needs based on relevant data (such as a high proportion of specific diagnostic groups such as post-traumatic stress disorder in some areas; percentage of older people; or the number of psychoactive substance abusers). Resources are then distributed through special programmes on a yearly basis.

Denmark's five regions usually take into account the proportions of various population groups in their local area as part of their mental health care planning.

In the Russian Federation, the allocation of funds takes into account the total number of adults and children, the total health budget in the region and several other parameters.

Only a few countries indicate that the budget allocation takes into account multiple indicators: in the United Kingdom (England and Wales), funding is distributed using complex needs formulas. Services are then commissioned locally based on detailed local needs assessment.

Main activities initiated or developed since 2005 related to funding of mental health services

- Ireland: A vision for change acknowledges that substantial extra funding is required to finance implementation (about €150 million). Additional funding of €51 million was provided in 2006 and 2007. A vision for change recommends that capital and human resources be remodelled and that funds raised from the sale of lands attached to former psychiatric hospitals be used to finance the development of mental health services (such as community-based mental health services).
- Latvia: financing for reconstruction and development of mental health facilities in regions (including mental hospitals) is a priority. The mental health system is one of the most important priorities in EU-funded programmes. New policy draft documents indicate money for the development of community care (outpatient clinics and community residential facilities).
- United Kingdom (Scotland): Delivering for Mental Health targets reducing the use of antidepressants and initiatives to increase the use of psychological interventions by 2010.

Table 8.5. Allocation of the local or regional budget for mental health care based on a formula taking into account the relative needs of the population in groups of countries

Allocation taking account of the population's needs	EU		EU15		New EU countries since 2004		Israel, Norway and Switzerland		South-eastern Europe		CIS		Total	
	No.	%	No.	%	No.	%	No.	%	No.	%	No.	%	No.	%
Yes	9	33	8	53	1	8	0	0	2	29	1	20	12	29
No	17	63	7	47	10	83	0	0	1	14	3	60	21	50
Information not available	1	4	0	0	1	8	3	100	4	57	1	20	9	21

Discussion

This chapter addresses the investment in mental health, the distribution of funding and equitability of access. It provides some important information, partly by the presence of data and partly by its absence.

Table 8.1 and Fig. 8.1 on the proportion of the health budget allocated to mental health show a familiar variation in distribution, with higher-income countries spending higher proportions on mental health. Since higher-income countries also generally invest a higher proportion of their gross domestic product in health, the effect is that spending on mental health is much higher in the EU15 countries, especially compared with south-eastern Europe and CIS countries. This is reflected in the complex mental health systems developed in some of the EU15 countries, as described in the earlier chapter on services. It also might explain the lack of services in the countries with fewer resources. Implementing and delivering community-based services on a very low budget is challenging. Countries with low spending on mental health such as Portugal and Bulgaria might be struggling to implement reforms, and higher investment seems necessary. Countries with high mental health spending tend to invest lower proportions of their budget on mental hospital care.

These national figures do not take into account local spending, particularly on community services and social care, which are often the responsibility of regional or local governments, whereas mental hospitals are often a national responsibility. The lack of disaggregation of mental health budgets in most countries and the inability to identify local spending on mental health services is one of the consequences of decentralization of provision, offering only a partial picture. It may mean that real spending on mental health care is much higher than national budget figures indicate.

Few countries provide figures on spending on promoting mental health and preventing mental disorders, but the data available are consistently very low, at most about 1% of the mental health budget. This is surprising, considering the richness of initiatives identified in previous chapters. Many such initiatives may be small scale and funded by local or independent funding sources, such as employers. Considering the centrality of mental health promotion and mental disorder prevention to policy-making in response to the high burden resulting from mental health problems and their high profile in the Mental Health Declaration for Europe and EU policy activities, this is an area that deserves close scrutiny for opportunities for effective investment.

Quite consistently, medication was available free of charge or fully reimbursed for people with severe mental health problems, particularly in hospital settings, which was 100% covered. Community and primary care settings showed high coverage but greater variation. Some countries distinguished along diagnostic lines, with such disorders as schizophrenia always qualifying for free reimbursement but depression in some countries requiring co-payment. All countries use some form of means testing, exempting the poorest and most vulnerable people from payment. However, the survey also identified that medication free of charge cannot always be guaranteed due to supply problems. In some of the lower-income countries, a limited quantity of medication was available free of charge, and once exhausted, people are expected to pay themselves. For some medication, this could imply a substantial part of their income. It could also easily result in abuse.

Access and reimbursement to psychotherapy is quite strictly controlled in some countries and not always available, particularly in primary care. This is ironic, considering the evidence of its cost-effectiveness and lack of side effects. Some countries are now actively investing in increasing their capacity to address needs in this area, particularly by training staff in cognitive behavioural therapy.

The distribution of funding determines the equitable allocation to vulnerable areas, groups and individuals. Funding formulas may produce such a distribution on an objective basis, incorporating weighting for factors such as the age of the population, socioeconomic deprivation, unemployment and ethnic minority groups. Few countries apply such formulas. Instead distribution seems to be based on historical allocation or more informal allocation arrangements. Countries could exchange experiences in this field.

Some serious challenges remain. First, much information is lacking altogether or lacks precision. Much of the data in this chapter are indicative, collected in different ways, but also including and excluding various variables. Numerators and denominators are not always identical. Specific data about local government investment in social care, including residential facilities, are very rarely reliably collected.

A second problem running throughout this report is that countries have different health and social care systems and are at very different stages of development. What is meant by investment in certain areas and on what the money is being spent are not always clear.

The lack of transparency about some of the data and the absence of so much detail raise questions about governance. If countries really have such few data on spending, how is effectiveness judged and how are future investment decisions decided? This theme re-emerges in Chapter 11 (on information and research). This is a great challenge for the future activities of WHO and the further implementation of the Mental Health Declaration for Europe and Mental Health Action Plan for Europe.

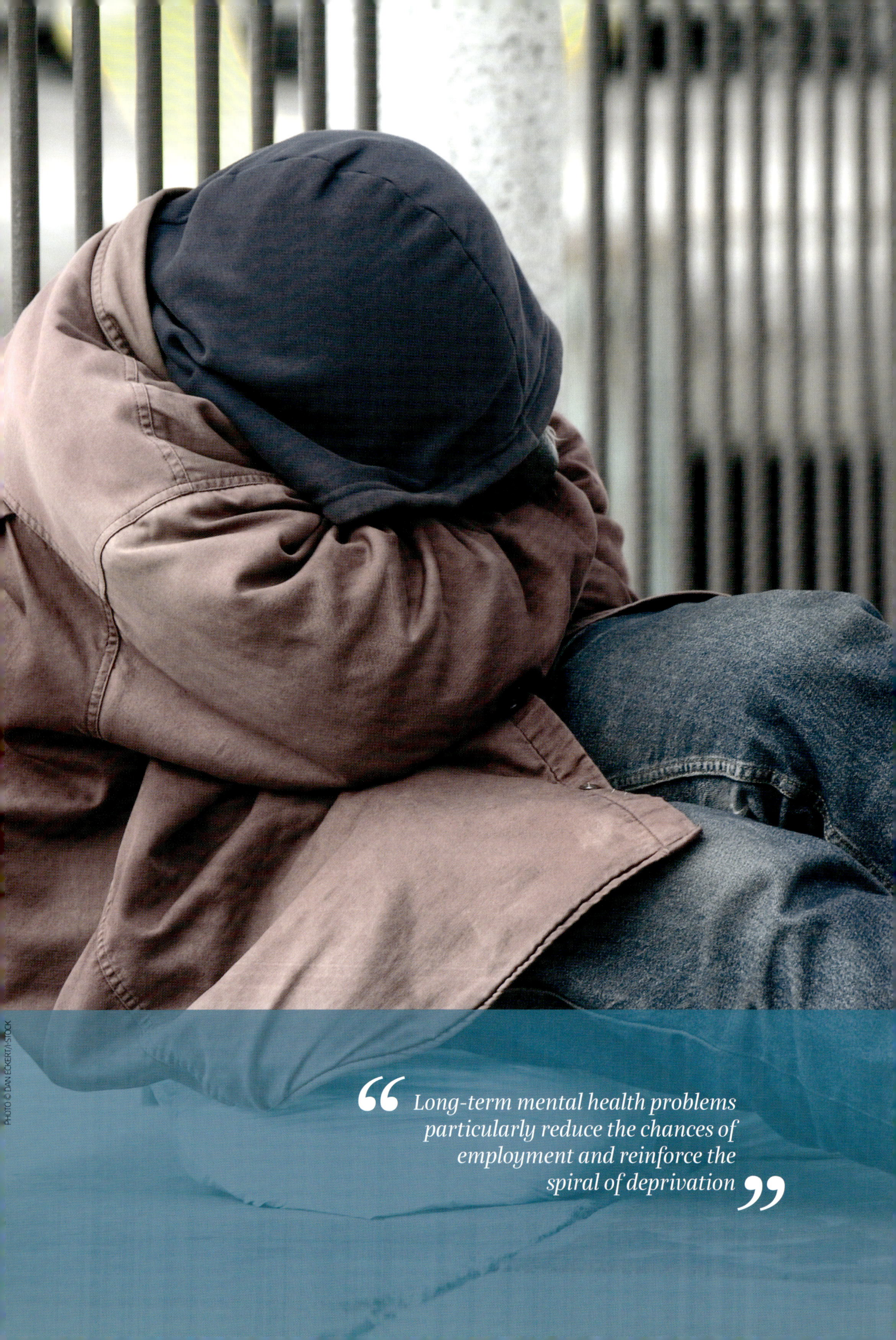

PHOTO © DAN ECKERT/ISTOCK

"Long-term mental health problems particularly reduce the chances of employment and reinforce the spiral of deprivation"

9. Social inclusion and welfare

People with mental health problems are at high risk of social exclusion due to a variety of factors. They encounter discrimination in all areas of their life: from accessing employment, health care, education, housing, social security and public services to the justice system, their communities and social networks, home life and personal and intimate relationships. Many live in housing or institutions identified with mental illness and are therefore avoided by members of communities. The negative consequences of their disorders can result in disability, including self-imposed stigma and discrimination. Social inclusion is recognized as a key issue on the political agenda of decision-makers in health and other sectors, especially in the EU countries.

Intervention by governments is therefore crucial to enhance the quality of life and social inclusion and stop stigma and discrimination.

Definition

For the purposes of this project, social inclusion has been defined as the process that ensures that those at risk of poverty and social exclusion gain the opportunities and resources necessary to participate fully in economic, social and cultural life and to enjoy a standard of living and well-being that is considered normal in the society in which they live.

Such interventions are not effective if they only target health. They need to encompass all the areas that have the potential to contribute to inclusion in the community, especially those that will support an integrated and decent life such as housing, employment and a fair income. All these need to be grounded on protection from discrimination. A particular

Fig. 9.1. Proportion of people receiving social welfare benefits or pensions because of disability due to mental health problems in countries

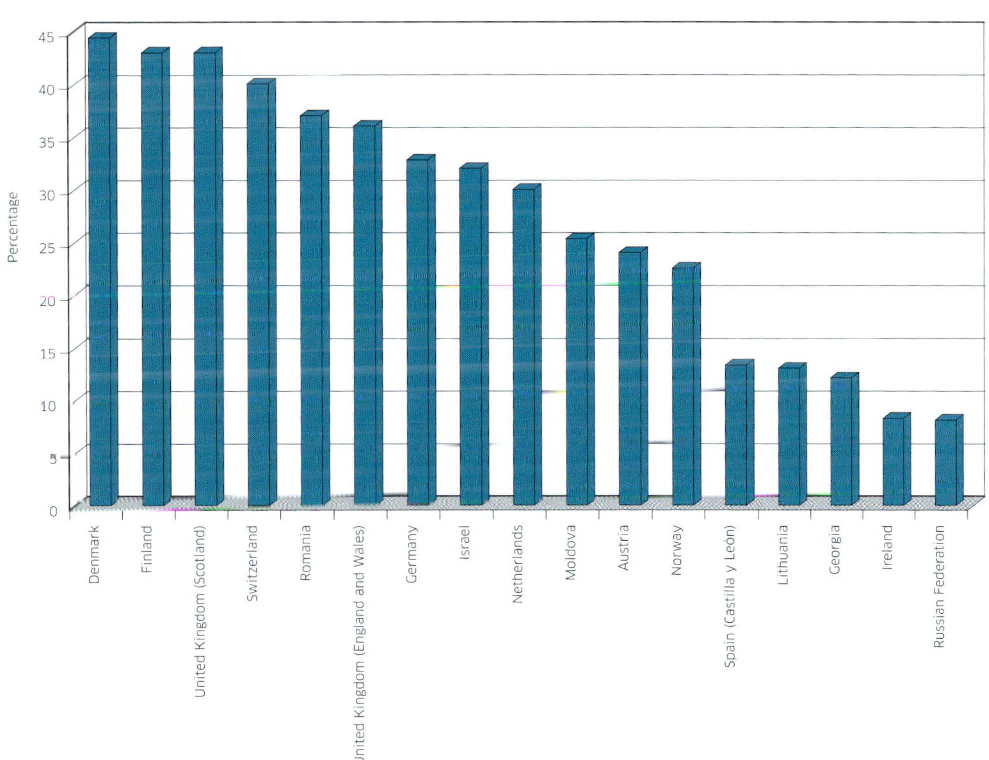

challenge is how to distinguish between policies that exclusively target the needs of people with mental health problems and those that aim to support all people with disabilities, focusing on integration.

Social welfare benefits or pensions because of disability due to mental health problems

The importance of addressing the consequences of disability caused by mental health problems is powerfully made when the contribution of mental disorders to the burden of disability is considered (Fig. 9.1). Data on the proportion of disabled people who are receiving social welfare benefits or pensions as a consequence of mental health problems are available for 17 of 42 countries. The countries for which data are available report proportions ranging from 44% in Denmark to 8% in the Russian Federation. The lack of data in other countries can be explained because the social care authorities or institutions responsible for people with all disabilities are responsible for welfare benefits and pensions.

Due to the complexity and diversity of social welfare systems, data are not always directly comparable across countries.

Mental illness as a cause of sick leave

Information on mental illness as a cause of sick leave is available for 16 of 42 countries, and the variation is by more than 10 times (Fig. 9.2). The very large differences between

Fig. 9.2. Proportion of people on sick leave due to mental illness during the last available year in countries

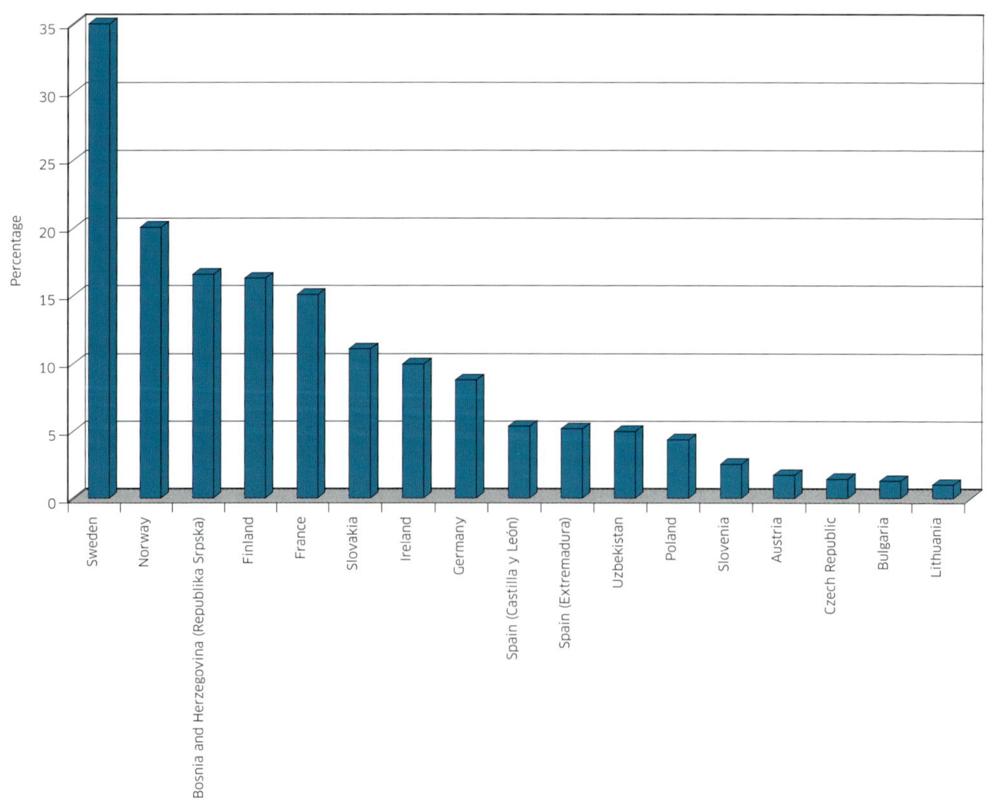

neighbouring countries such as Sweden and Norway and the very low rates in countries such as Austria and especially Lithuania suggest that several factors may explain the variation and hinder comparability, such as validity of recording, but also possibly legal reasons and stigma.

There are very different reasons why data on the causes of sick leave are not available. In Denmark, Italy and the Russian Federation, such information is confidential and legislation does not allow specification. In France, the cause of sick leave does not have to be justified. In Portugal, the data exist but are difficult to collect from the authorities responsible for collecting this information.

Policies and programmes to improve social inclusion

Most countries address this area, indicating the general acceptance that people with mental health problems are at risk of social exclusion and discrimination. Of the 42 countries, 34 (81%) have either policies or programmes aimed at increasing the level of social inclusion for people with mental health problems, very consistently across all groups of countries, although the ambition and scope of programmes differ (Box 9.1). Far fewer countries have introduced legislative procedures solely to protect people with mental health problems. The benefits of such exclusive measures can only be judged in the context of the needs of people with mental health problems and already available general rights.

Box 9.1. Social inclusion programmes in the United Kingdom (England and Wales)

SHIFT is part of the Care Services Improvement Partnership, a government-funded organization that supports positive changes in services and in the well-being of vulnerable people with health and social care needs. SHIFT is a five-year initiative (2004–2009) in England to tackle stigma and discrimination surrounding mental health issues. The work is set out in a plan called From Here to Equality. SHIFT's aim is to create a society in which people who experience mental health problems enjoy the same rights as other people. To work towards this, SHIFT works with young people, public services, private, voluntary and professional organizations and the mass media, drawing on expertise in public health and mental health promotion, communications, disability rights, service redesign, research and evaluation. SHIFT builds on the mind out for mental health campaign, which ran from 2001 to April 2004.

The Care Services Improvement Partnership is working to offer more choice to all people who use mental health services. The Our Choices in Mental Health programme continues to explore how people who use mental health services and their carers can exercise more choice over their treatment and care. It provides a best-practice framework for providers to extend choices, practical support and examples of service models from across England.

The Improving Access to Psychological Therapies programme seeks to deliver on the government's 2005 general election manifesto commitment to provide improved access to psychological therapy for people who require the help of mental health services. It also responds to service user's requests for more personalized services based on their individual needs. It will test the effectiveness of providing increases in evidence-based psychological therapy services to people with "common" mental health problems such as anxiety and depression, in providing improvements in health, well-being and in maintaining people or returning people to employment and community participation. The programme has two national demonstration sites, in Newham and Doncaster, and a national network of local psychological therapy programmes in each of the eight Care Services Improvement Partnership regional development centres.

Box 9.1. continued

The Whole Life Programme is led by the Eastern Development Centre of the Care Services Improvement Partnership, working in partnership with the South West Development Centre since 2003. There are now 11 development sites and systems linked to the Whole Life Programme, and close links are being established with the National Social Inclusion Programme. The overall aim of the Whole Life Programme is to ensure that local service delivery can more closely reflect the needs and aims of individual service users in all their dimensions and provide a much more person-centred, holistic empowering response involving a growing range of mainstream resources in local communities as well as local statutory and independent service providers. The programme focuses particularly on establishing a more explicit and appropriate value base for those working at all levels in local services and ensuring that this is put into operation at all levels of the system from the strategic vision set by commissioners and senior managers through the work of individual practitioners working in frontline services. It is believed that changing the thinking of practitioners, managers and service users will influence practice and provide a powerful driver for system reform and responsive services. A Whole Life value base essentially reflects the principles advocated in the overlapping agendas around user and carer involvement, social inclusion, recovery, values into practice, individualized budgets, choice, outcomes, development of new community services and service improvement.

Mental health promotion: Standard One of the National Service Framework for Mental Health states that health and social services should: promote mental health for all, working with individuals and communities; and combat discrimination against individuals and groups with mental health problems and promote their social inclusion. Many people working locally have felt a sense of isolation in advocating for mental health promotion. To help address this, the National Institute for Mental Health in England is bringing together a national Mental Health Promotion Advisory Group, whose chief aims are:

- to raise the national profile of the commitment in Standard One of the National Service Framework for Mental Health: "to promote mental health for all, working with individuals, organizations and communities";
- to support Goal 2 in the National Suicide Prevention Strategy – "To promote mental well-being in the wider population" – as part of the effort to reduce deaths from suicide and undetermined injury by 20% by 2010;
- to assemble and disseminate evidence of effective interventions in promoting the mental health of the whole population at the national, regional and local levels;
- to develop resources to support the work of Standard One leads at the regional and local levels;
- to establish baseline measures of the mental health of the population and/or its known determinants and a method for monitoring progress;
- to work with the Department of Health and other government departments on the wider determinants of mental health, in the context of the Wanless report Securing good health for the whole population, the public health consultation Choosing Health and Tackling Health Inequalities: a Programme for Action.

Table 9.1. Presence of legislative provisions on protection from discrimination (housing, dismissal and lower wages) solely because of mental disorder in groups of countries

Legal protection from discrimination	EU		EU15		New EU countries since 2004		Israel, Norway and Switzerland		South-eastern Europe		CIS		Total	
	No.	%	No.	%	No.	%	No.	%	No.	%	No.	%	No.	%
Legislative or financial provisions														
Enforced	13	48	10	67	3	25	2	67	3	43	2	40	20	48
Not enforced	6	22	1	7	5	42	1	33	0	0	2	40	9	21
Legislation or financial provisions being planned	1	4	0	0	1	8	0	0	0	0	0	0	1	2
No legislation or financial provisions	7	26	4	27	3	25	0	0	4	57	1	20	12	29

It is not always known whether these programmes have the intended impact, since few have been evaluated. Examples of programmes aiming to increase social inclusion are:

- Finland: fountain houses (from 1998 to the present) and Law on Social Enterprises (1351/2003).
- Georgia: State Program of Social Integration for Disabled People (including people with mental disabilities), 2006–2007.
- Ireland: A vision for change (7–10 years).
- Italy: projects related to the EQUAL Initiative funded by the European Social Fund.
- Latvia: EQUAL Initiative project on integration of people with mental disturbances and mental illnesses in the labour market; work for mental health service users; integration into the labour market; support in the workplace; assessment (2005–2007).
- Netherlands: protected employment for 100 000 people with disability, including chronic mental health problems. This is an ongoing programme initiated 50 years ago.
- Sweden: mental health care reform (1995–1998).
- Stability Pact for South Eastern Europe countries: South-eastern Europe Mental Health Project from 2003 to the present.

Legal protection from discrimination: housing, dismissal and lower wages

Anti-discrimination legislation covering housing, dismissal and lower wages has been adopted and enforced in 20 of 42 countries (Table 9.1). Such legislation is typically aimed at protecting all the people with disability (including those with mental disorders) from unfair treatment solely on account of their disability. This includes 10 of the EU15 countries and 3 of the 12 countries that have joined the EU since 2004. Another nine countries indicated that, although legislation has been adopted, it is not enforced.

Some countries have dedicated anti-discrimination legislation with clear mechanisms for implementation and have assigned institutions in charge of overseeing their enforcement.

- In Ireland, the Employment Equality Act 1998, the Equal Status Act 2000 and the Equality Act 2004 provide legislative protection against discrimination in employment and in the provision of goods and services. The Department of Justice, Equality and Law Reform is responsible for these acts. They define disability as (a) the total or partial absence of a person's bodily or mental functions, including the absence of a part of a person's body, (b) the presence in the body of organisms causing, or likely to cause, chronic disease or illness, (c) the malfunction, malformation or disfigurement of part of a person's body, (d) a condition or malfunction that results in a person learning differently from a person without the condition or malfunction or (e) a condition, illness or disease that affects a person's thought processes, perception of reality, emotions or judgement or that results in disturbed behaviour, and shall be taken to include a disability that exists at present or that previously existed but no longer exists or that may exist in the future or that is imputed to a person.

- In Romania, legislation on protection against discrimination was adopted in 2000 (Government Ordinance No. 137/2000 on preventing and penalizing all forms of discrimination), and a National Council for Combating Discrimination has been established to monitor the enforcement of the legislation. The Council has the means and capacity to pursue cases of discrimination and has done so in some health and non-health areas. So far no case of discrimination has been filed on mental grounds.
- In the United Kingdom (England and Wales), the Disability Discrimination Act 2005 includes some groups of people with mental disorders. It provides protection from discrimination in employment and in the provision of goods and services.
- In Germany's labour law, no regulations have been adopted for specific protection against discrimination because of mental illness. Mental disorders are treated in the same way as physical illnesses. Hence, according to the Continuation of Wage Payments Act, people suffering from mental disorders are entitled to the continued payment of wages in cases of occupational disability for which they are not at fault, or in the wake of illness, regardless of the type of illness. The Protection against Dismissal Act also makes no differentiation between physical and mental illness regarding the social justification of the termination of employment because of illness. In addition, legal provisions regulate the specific protection against unfair termination for severely disabled people. Here, again, the severity of the disability and not the type of disability is decisive (General Equal Treatment Act and the Severely Disabled Persons Act in Volume 9 of the Social Code, Part 2).

In other countries (such as Georgia and Italy), measures for protecting against discrimination are incorporated into various legislative documents addressing employment, social protection, etc.

Adopting legislation does not guarantee that people with mental health problems are protected against discrimination. It is doubtful that the following two examples are exclusive.

- Georgia has no such separate legislation or other provisions. The Law on Psychiatric Care refers to patients' social protection and right to education and retraining. Article 5 notes that the patient is entitled to enjoy all rights provided under the legislation of Georgia. Article 6 reads: "Restriction of patient's rights solely on the basis of mental disorder is inadmissible. Any kind of restriction determined by Georgian legislation should be based not only on the diagnosis of mental disorder but on the mental health state of person and the level of his/her social adaptation." However, in reality people with mental disorders suffer discrimination, since they cannot receive relevant and high-quality health care; their rights to education, employment and provision of living space are infringed. The present system of mental health care cannot ensure their effective treatment and reintegration into society.
- In Lithuania, legislative provisions on protection from discrimination are implemented in the law on mental health care, in the law on social integration of people with disabilities and the law on equal opportunities. But in real life discrimination does take place.

Subsidized housing for people with severe mental disorders

People with severe mental disorders are entitled to subsidized housing in 28 of 42 countries, including 12 of the EU15 countries and 8 of the 12 countries joining the EU since May 2004 (Table 9.2). Legislation guaranteeing this entitlement is not enforced in five of these countries. Further, two countries (both EU) report that plans are currently under development for legislation or financial provisions.

Table 9.2. Presence of legislative or financial provisions on subsidized housing for people with severe mental disorders in groups of countries

Legislative or financial support for subsidized housing	EU		EU15		New EU countries since 2004		Israel, Norway and Switzerland		South-eastern Europe		CIS		Total	
	No.	%	No.	%	No.	%	No.	%	No.	%	No.	%	No.	%
Legislative or financial provisions														
Enforced	18	67	11	73	7	58	3	100	0	0	2	40	23	55
Not enforced	2	7	1	7	1	8	0	0	2	29	1	20	5	12
Legislation or financial provisions being planned	2	7	1	7	1	8	0	0	0	0	0	0	2	5
No legislation or financial provisions	5	19	2	13	3	25	0	0	5	71	2	40	12	29

The meaning of subsidized housing differs across the WHO European Region. In most of the EU countries, it refers to financial support for people with severe disorders to cover housing expenses, protected houses, shelters, hostels and other forms of integrated living.

- Austria: rules differ for each province; for example, Styria has legislative and financial provisions (the law includes a definition of several types of subsidized housing; people with mental disorders who comply with the requirements have the right to obtain the accommodation needed).
- France: people with long-term mental disability can benefit from different forms of housing adapted to their needs, on a temporary or a long-term basis. There are more medicalized solutions for highly dependent people (specialized welcoming houses and medical hostels). Act No. 2007 290 of 5 March 2007 instituting the right to housing and providing for diverse measures supporting social cohesion guarantees the right to healthy and independent housing by the state to any person permanently living in France who cannot access it on his or her own or cannot stay there.
- United Kingdom (England and Wales): local authorities provide housing benefit to people on low incomes to assist with their rental payments. People with severe and enduring mental health problems are a large proportion of the groups claiming incapacity benefit and as such would also be claiming housing benefit.

In countries in the eastern part of the WHO European Region (such as Azerbaijan and Uzbekistan), subsidized housing refers to social institutions where people with severe disorders, once admitted, usually live for the rest of their lives.

Some of the countries joining the EU since 2004 and countries in south-eastern Europe are in the process of transition between large institutions with poor living conditions and a minimal level of health care to a modern model of protected housing and financial support for independent living. This is reported to be the case in Albania, Bosnia and Herzegovina and Romania, albeit at a very small scale. The health sector has initiated pilot initiatives, often benefiting from international funding. At the same time, the social sector is increasingly active in several countries that joined the EU after 2004 (such as Lithuania and Romania), although this remains largely disconnected from initiatives in the health sector.

Supported employment for people who are disabled due to mental disorders

Legislative or financial incentives for employers to hire employees that are disabled due to mental disorders have been adopted in 28 of 42 countries (67%) and are implemented in 23 of the 42 countries (55%). These provisions are reportedly adopted and enforced in 10 of the EU15 countries, 6 of the 12 countries joining the EU since 2004, 2 of the 5 CIS countries and 3 of the 7 countries in south-eastern Europe (Table 9.3).

Table 9.3. Presence of legislative or financial provisions for employers to hire employees who are disabled due to mental disorders in groups of countries

Legislative or financial support employment	EU		EU15		New EU countries since 2004		Israel, Norway and Switzerland		South-eastern Europe		CIS		Total	
	No.	%	No.	%	No.	%	No.	%	No.	%	No.	%	No.	%
Legislative or financial provisions														
Enforced	16	59	10	67	6	50	2	67	3	43	2	40	23	55
Not enforced	3	11	2	13	1	8	0	0	2	29	0	0	5	12
Legislation or financial provisions being planned	2	7	0	0	2	17	0	0	0	0	1	20	3	7
No legislation or financial provisions	6	22	3	20	3	25	1	33	2	29	2	40	11	26

While 11 of 42 countries indicate that no such legislation provisions exist, 3 countries (Cyprus, Moldova and Slovakia) noted that they are currently planning to develop such legal initiatives.

The following are specific country examples.

- Austria: the Behinderteneinstellungsgesetz (Federal Disability Equality Act). In practice, it is easier for people with physical disability to obtain a job than for people with mental disorders, similar to other countries; a company may also be fined for not employing a person with disability.
- Bulgaria: the employers receive financial incentives to hire people with mental health disability. There is a Law on Integration of the People with Disabilities (including mental disability). The part on employment, §24–27, describes the conditions for hiring people with long-term disability by regular employers. There is also a registry of specialized companies and enterprises where people with (mental) disability can be hired. The Agency for People with Disabilities maintains the registry. Other relevant regulations such as the Labour Code and Law for Protection, Rehabilitation and Social Integration of Disabled People have stipulations about these opportunities.
- Germany: in general, if employers employ 20 people or more, at least 5% of the employees are required to be people with severe disability. This means, however, that the severity and not the type of disability plays a role. There are no regulations of this type that apply only to people with mental disorders.

  Related laws: Volume 9 of the Social Code – Rehabilitation and Participation; the Obligation to Employ Disabled Persons, Article 72. Employment of special groups of severely disabled people:

  (1) Within the framework of fulfilling the obligation to employ disabled people, the following groups are to be employed in appropriate measure:
    a. severely disabled people, who are extremely disadvantaged in working life due to their disabilities, especially those who: a) require a long-term special assistant to perform their work because of their disability; or b) whose employment as a result of their disability is not only temporarily connected with unusual expense for the employer; or c) who, as a result of their disability, are obviously appreciably less productive for longer than just a temporary period; or d) for whom a degree of disability of at least 50% results from intellectual or mental disorder or from seizures; or e) who, because of the type or degree of their disability, have never completed vocational training as defined by the Vocational Training Act; and
    b. severely disabled people over 50 years of age.

  (2) employers with places for occupational training, especially apprentices, shall place an appropriate proportion of disabled people in these places within

the framework of the fulfilment of their obligation to employ disabled people.

- Switzerland: financial support and advice to employers about hiring people with health-related restrictions on their performance (including that determined by mental disorders). The 5th Revision of the Disability Insurance Act that entered into force on 1 January 2008 includes integration measures that are available for mentally ill people in particular. These integration measures are intended to bring mentally ill people back into the world of work in the context of "supported employment". Employers receive financial support for this as well as targeted coaching.

Formal collaborative programmes between mental health departments and agencies and other parts of the health sector and other sectors

Countries were asked to assess the interagency cooperation aimed at increasing the level of support offered to people with mental health problems and at facilitating their social inclusion.

Partnerships within the health sector

Within the health care sector, information was collected about partnerships between the department or agency responsible for mental health and:

- primary health care and community health
- HIV and AIDS
- reproductive health
- child and adolescent health
- substance misuse.

The most frequent partnership is between mental health and substance misuse – 33 of 42 countries (79%) report formal collaborative programmes (Table 9.4).

In contrast, partnerships with departments or agencies responsible for reproductive health have been established in 13 of 42 countries (31%).

The partnership with primary health care and community health is crucial to ensure the continuity of care after discharge from specialist services. Such collaborative programmes are in place in 11 of the EU15 countries (73%) versus only 6 of the 12 countries that joined the EU since 2004 (50%). None of the CIS countries report such partnerships.

The following sections show some examples of partnerships. Note the high number of partnership initiatives that rely on funding and delivery by external agencies.

Primary health care and community health

- Bosnia and Herzegovina (Republika Srpska): cooperation between centres for mental health and the Red Cross in municipal programmes to offer support in social care, which includes people with mental health problems. Cooperation with nongovernmental organizations in some specific educational projects for young people.
- Czech Republic: the Centre for Mental Health Care Development is responsible for educating GPs.
- Georgia: preparation of family doctors for diagnosing some types of mental disorders and their management only; however, this has not been introduced in practice yet.
- United Kingdom (England and Wales): The National Social Inclusion Programme links with the Improving Access to Psychological Therapies primary care programme through workforce development.
- United Kingdom (Scotland): programmes are in place in local agencies to address the needs of people with mental illness in a variety of settings.

HIV and AIDS

- Bosnia and Herzegovina: cooperation with mental health centres in a project for preventing sexually transmitted infections, supported by the Association for Sexual and Reproductive Health XY (a nongovernmental organization) and the United Nations Population Fund (UNFPA).
- Russian Federation: with the Ministry of Education (HIV prevention in educational institutions) and Ministry of Justice (HIV prevention in the penitentiary system) – there is no comprehensive national programme, and the activities are at interinstitutional level.

Table 9.4. Formal collaborative programmes addressing the needs of people with mental health issues between the department or agency responsible for mental health and others within the health sector in countries

Country	Primary health care and community health	HIV and AIDS	Reproductive health	Adolescent health	Substance abuse
Albania	No	No	No	No	Yes
Austria	No	No	No	No	No
Azerbaijan	No	No	No	No	No
Belgium	Yes	Information not available	Information not available	Yes	Yes
Bosnia and Herzegovina					
Federation of Bosnia and Herzegovina	Yes	Yes	Yes	Yes	Yes
Republika Srpska	Yes	Yes	Yes	Yes	Yes
Bulgaria	Yes	Yes	Yes	Yes	Yes
Croatia	Yes	No	Yes	Yes	Yes
Cyprus	No	No	No	Yes	Yes
Czech Republic	Yes	Information not available	Information not available	Information not available	Yes
Denmark	Yes	No	Yes	Yes	Yes
Estonia	No	Yes	No	Yes	Yes
Finland	Yes	Information not available	Information not available	Yes	Yes
France	Yes	Yes	Information not available	Yes	Yes
Georgia	No	Yes	No	No	No
Germany	Yes	Yes	Information not available	Yes	Yes
Greece	Yes	No	No	Yes	Yes
Hungary	No	Yes	No	Yes	Yes
Ireland	Information not available	Information not available	Information not available	Information not available	Information not available
Israel	No	No	No	Yes	Yes
Italy	Yes	Yes	Yes	Yes	Yes
Latvia	No	No	No	No	No
Lithuania	Yes	Yes	Information not available	Yes	Yes
Luxembourg	Yes	Yes	Yes	Yes	Yes
Malta	Yes	No	Yes	Yes	Yes
Moldova	No	No	No	Yes	Yes
Montenegro	Information not available	Yes	Information not available	Information not available	Yes
Netherlands	Yes	Yes	Yes	Yes	Yes
Norway	Yes	Information not available	Yes	Yes	Yes
Poland	Yes	Yes	Information not available	Yes	Yes
Portugal	No	No	No	No	No
Romania	Yes	No	No	Yes	Yes
Russian Federation	Information not available	Yes	Information not available	Yes	Yes
Serbia	Yes	Yes	Yes	Yes	Yes
Slovakia	Information not available	No	No	Information not available	No
Slovenia	No	No	No	Yes	Yes
Spain					
Castilla y León	Yes	No	No	Yes	Yes
Catalonia	Yes	Yes	Yes	Yes	Yes
Extremadura	Yes	Information not available	Information not available	Information not available	Yes
Galicia	Yes	No	Yes	Yes	Yes
Murcia	Yes	No	No	Yes	Yes
Sweden	Information not available	Information not available	Information not available	Information not available	Information not available
Switzerland	No	No	No	Yes	Yes
The former Yugoslav Republic of Macedonia	No	No	No	No	No
Turkey	Yes	Yes	Information not available	Yes	Yes
United Kingdom					
England and Wales	Yes	Yes	Yes	Yes	Yes
Scotland	Yes	Information not available	Information not available	Information not available	Information not available
Uzbekistan	No	Yes	Yes	Yes	Yes

Yes / No / Information not available

- Serbia: United Nations Development Programme (UNDP) programme with local nongovernmental organization and the Ministry of Health – Global Fund to Fight AIDS, Tuberculosis and Malaria programme.
- Spain (Catalonia): special units for mental health and AIDS.
- Uzbekistan: National AIDS Centre programme funded by the Global Fund to Fight AIDS, Tuberculosis and Malaria for psychological support of people living with HIV and preventing depression. A manual on telephone psychological counselling was published in 2005.

Child and adolescent health

- Belgium: the centres for student counselling make formal agreements with the mental health centres in their region (Flemish Government).
- Russian Federation: with the Ministry of Education; within the Federal Programme "Children of Russia", implementation of an anti-drug prevention programme in institutions for children and adolescents (schools, education and leisure centres); specialist training for professionals in education and mental health. Introduction of an integrative approach for a healthy environment for children by municipal education departments.
- Uzbekistan: WHO/UNICEF programme on child development and joint programme of the Cabinet of Ministers and Women's Committee on family education for children younger than five years including the mental development of children.

Partnerships between the health sector and other sectors

Countries were asked to provide information on partnerships in place between the mental health sector and other sectors (Table 9.5):

- education
- employment
- housing
- welfare
- child protection
- older people
- criminal justice
- other departments and agencies.

More than half the countries have partnership programmes in place between the department or agency responsible for mental health and the education, welfare, child protection, older people and criminal justice sectors, although many programmes are small scale and local.

Partnerships with the employment sector have been established in 43% of the countries, including 73% of the EU15 countries but only 33% of the countries that joined the EU since 2004, 14% of the countries in south-eastern Europe and no CIS country.

Another important partnership, that with the housing sector, is in place in only 16 of 42 countries: 67% of the EU15 countries, 25% of the countries that joined the EU since 2004, 14% of the countries in south-eastern Europe and no CIS country.

Main activities initiated and developed since 2005 related to social inclusion and partnership

Social inclusion of people with mental health problems

Social inclusion activities

- Advocacy campaigns and a few pilot projects aiming to create income-generating activities or social activities (Albania).
- Activities aimed at supporting service users in finding appropriate daytime activities, such as work, education, leisure activities and meetings (Belgium).
- Inclusion programmes for children in special schools (Bosnia and Herzegovina (Federation of Bosnia and Herzegovina)) or regular schools (Bosnia and Herzegovina (Republika Srpska)).
- Activities focused on supported housing for people with psychotic disorders (Cyprus).
- Implementation of projects funded by the European Social Fund (Czech Republic and Latvia).
- Creation of mobile psychiatric teams (France); projects aimed at improving the integration of people with (mental) disability into the labour market and offering funding for people with mental disability (Germany).

Table 9.5. Formal collaborative programmes addressing the needs of people with mental health issues between the department or agency responsible for mental health and other sectors in countries

Country	Education	Employment	Housing	Welfare	Child protection	Older people	Criminal justice
Albania	Yes	Yes	Yes	Yes	No	No	Yes
Austria	No	No	No	No	No	No	No
Azerbaijan	No	No	No	No	No	No	No
Belgium	Yes	Information not available	Information not available	Yes	Yes	Yes	Yes
Bosnia and Herzegovina							
Federation of Bosnia and Herzegovina	Yes	No	No	Yes	Yes	No	Yes
Republika Srpska	Yes	No	No	Yes	Yes	Yes	Yes
Bulgaria	No	No	Yes	Yes	No	No	No
Croatia	Yes	No	No	Yes	Yes	Yes	Yes
Cyprus	Yes	No	No	Yes	Yes	No	Yes
Czech Republic	Yes	Information not available	Information not available	Information not available	Information not available	Information not available	Information not available
Denmark	Yes	Yes	Yes	Yes	Yes	Yes	Yes
Estonia	Yes	Yes	Yes	Yes	Yes	Yes	Yes
Finland	Yes	Yes	Yes	Yes	Yes	Yes	Yes
France	Yes	Yes	Yes	Information not available	Yes	Yes	Yes
Georgia	No	No	No	Yes	No	No	Yes
Germany	Yes	Yes	Yes	Yes	Yes	Yes	Yes
Greece	Yes	Yes	Information not available	Yes	Yes	Yes	Information not available
Hungary	Yes	No	No	Yes	Yes	No	No
Ireland	Information not available	Information not available	Information not available	Information not available	Information not available	Information not available	Information not available
Israel	Yes	No	No	Yes	Yes	Yes	Yes
Italy	Yes	Yes	Yes	Yes	Yes	Yes	Yes
Latvia	No	No	No	No	No	No	No
Lithuania	Yes	Yes	Information not available	Yes	Yes	Yes	Yes
Luxembourg	Yes	Yes	Yes	Yes	Yes	Yes	Yes
Malta	Yes	Yes	No	Yes	Yes	Yes	No
Moldova	No	No	Information not available	No	No	No	No
Montenegro	Information not available	Information not available	Information not available	Information not available	Information not available	Information not available	Information not available
Netherlands	Yes	Yes	Yes	Yes	Yes	Yes	Yes
Norway	Information not available	Yes	Yes	Yes	Yes	Information not available	Information not available
Poland	Yes	Yes	Yes	Yes	Information not available	Information not available	Yes
Portugal	No	Yes	Yes	Yes	No	No	Yes
Romania	Yes	No	No	Yes	Yes	Yes	Yes
Russian Federation	Yes	No	Information not available	No	No	Information not available	Yes
Serbia	Yes	No	No	No	Yes	Yes	Yes
Slovakia	Yes	No	No	No	Yes	Yes	Information not available
Slovenia	No	No	No	No	No	No	No
Spain							
Castilla y León	Yes	No	No	Yes	Yes	Yes	No
Catalonia	Yes	No	Yes	Yes	Yes	Yes	Yes
Extremadura	Information not available	Yes	Information not available	Information not available	Information not available	Information not available	Yes
Galicia	Yes	No	No	Yes	Yes	Yes	Yes
Murcia	Yes	Yes	No	Information not available	No	No	Yes
Sweden	Information not available	Information not available	Information not available	Information not available	Information not available	Information not available	Information not available
Switzerland	Yes	Yes	Yes	No	No	Yes	No
The former Yugoslav Republic of Macedonia	No	No	No	No	No	No	No
Turkey	Information not available	Information not available	Information not available	Information not available	Information not available	Information not available	Information not available
United Kingdom							
England and Wales	Yes	Yes	Yes	Yes	Yes	Yes	Yes
Scotland	Information not available	Information not available	Information not available	Information not available	Information not available	Information not available	Information not available
Uzbekistan	Yes	No	No	No	Yes	Yes	Yes

■ Yes ■ No ■ Information not available

- Increasing the places in community rehabilitation services and developing specific programmes for people with mental health problems in prisons (Spain (Catalonia)).
- Programmes aimed at supporting carers in facilitating the social reintegration of service users upon discharge (Spain (Castilla y León)).
- Development of a network of community mutual-help houses (Poland).

Social inclusion in policies

- Adoption of new legislation on social inclusion (Bulgaria).
- Inclusion of provisions in health legislation (Denmark).
- Adoption of policies on social inclusion and the integration of people with disabilities (Estonia, Georgia and Romania).
- Ensuring that social inclusion is reflected in current health policy (Norway) and mental health policy (Lithuania).

Other

- Establishment of a National Economic and Social Forum project team in 2006 to examine mental health and social inclusion (Ireland).
- Implementation of the South-eastern Europe Mental Health Project in nine countries in south-eastern Europe.
- Implementation of the National Social Inclusion Programme (United Kingdom (England and Wales)); delivering on the new social inclusion targets in the Closing the Opportunity Gap approach (United Kingdom (Scotland)).

Partnership for intersectoral working

Development of partnership projects

- Between the Ministry of Health, the Ministry of Civil Affairs, the Ministry of Human Rights and Refugees and governments of neighbouring countries on providing housing and other benefits for people with mental problems displaced during the war in the 1990s (Bosnia and Herzegovina (Federation of Bosnia and Herzegovina)).
- Activities on preventing violence among children and adolescents and needs assessment and awareness-raising programme for bullying in schools (Cyprus).
- Between the health sector and the Ministry of Education on depression among children (Malta).

Policy framework for partnerships

- The National Social Inclusion Programme is a cross-government (20 government departments) and interagency (50 affiliated organizations) Programme working in partnership to improve the life chances of people with severe mental health problems. Annual reports are available at http://www.socialinclusion.org.uk/resources/index.php?subid=55 (United Kingdom (England and Wales)).
- The Department of Health's Improving Access to Psychological Therapies programme is a cross-government and interagency programme working to support and help people recover from depression and anxiety. For further details, see http://www.mhchoice.csip.org.uk (United Kingdom (England and Wales)).

Discussion

The data in this chapter confirm the very high proportion of disability that can be attributed to mental disorders. Although registration varies across countries and is probably strongly influenced by differences in regulation, data are quite consistent. Mental health problems also contribute significantly to sick leave. In combination, this underlines the major influence of mental health problems on personal suffering, family burden, social activities, economic deprivation and the productivity of the workforce. Added to this are the consequences of stigma and discrimination that accompany the presence of any disability. However, long-term mental health problems particularly reduce the chances of employment and reinforce the spiral of deprivation, both materially and socially. This chapter shows that most countries recognize such social exclusion and are attempting to redress this.

A challenging question is whether disabilities should be addressed as a group or whether certain specific conditions result in such high risk of or severity of exclusion and discrimination that targeted action or interventions are necessary. Such action also needs to be designed carefully to prevent unintentional additional stigma and discrimination by singling out and separating already stigmatized groups. Most countries seem to have chosen an integrated approach: disability rights and legislation that are based on the level of disability and not on the condition. This chapter has provided few examples of targeted interventions.

Most countries appear to have put in place legislation that guaranteed financial support for housing or incentives to employ people with disability, especially in the EU. A concern is that these entitlements are not always enforced and especially that people with mental health problems may be disproportionately excluded from employment opportunities. Further work on equitable access and the effectiveness of scrutiny will be worthwhile.

Mental health problems are strongly associated with wider social problems, either as cause or effect. Multi-agency partnerships are therefore vital. There are many formal arrangements between mental health and other health departments and agencies and between mental health agencies and other sectors, especially in the EU. There are some worrying gaps, such as partnerships with the employment, housing and welfare sectors. Of added concern is that some of the arrangements are very local and small scale, especially in the eastern part of the WHO European Region, where nongovernmental organizations fund and deliver many initiatives. This raises questions about sustainability and diffusion. The gap between some of the universal programmes in western EU countries and the local pilot programmes in other countries is striking.

The tremendous variety and creativity of initiatives in all the countries is positive, even though many are small scale. There is great diversity and great enthusiasm, which offers much scope for sharing and learning.

Finally, this chapter again demonstrates the importance of collecting consistent information. Although some conclusions can be made with confidence, more precise comparisons are very unreliable due to the variation in concepts and differences in the collection of information.

"There is a strong correlation between trends in mental health expenditure, trends in the development of community mental health services and the involvement of users and carers"

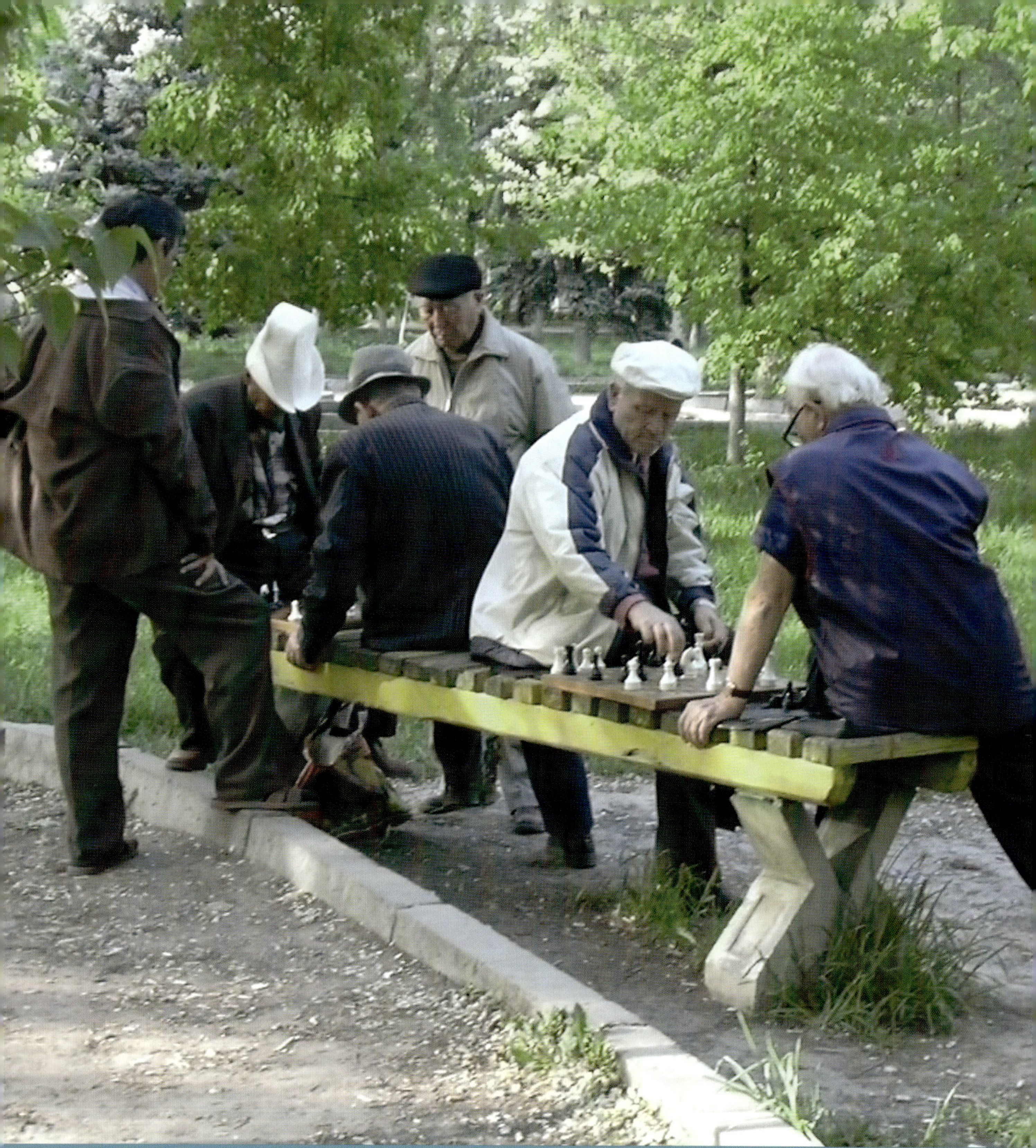

> “It would be of particular interest to determine the influence of groups of service users and carers on policy and practice”

10. Opportunities for the empowerment and representation of service users and carers

The Mental Health Declaration for Europe and Mental Health Action Plan for Europe identify the empowerment of service users and carers as one of the key priorities for the next decade. Specifically, Member States should work to recognize the experience and knowledge of service users and carers and use this experience as an important basis for planning and developing mental health services. Many of the areas for action explicitly state the importance of the contribution by users and carers, and the empowerment of users and carers is also a cross-cutting theme in both the Mental Health Declaration for Europe and the Mental Health Action Plan for Europe. Users and carers can contribute unique insights based on their personal experiences, which complement the expertise of planners, academics and providers and can help to ensure that services are designed to be efficient, effective and acceptable to users. This recognition reflects the experience of other sectors such as industry that consumer views must be reflected in product development and in continuous quality assurance – there is a moral, practical and business case for user empowerment. In addition, user empowerment has a therapeutic role for the individual.

Member States assumed responsibility to deliver on this priority at the national level and committed themselves to offering people with mental health problems choice and involvement in their own care, sensitive to their needs and culture and to support nongovernmental organizations active in the mental health field and stimulate the creation of nongovernmental and service user organizations. Echoing these commitments, the WHO European Member States agreed in the Mental Health Action Plan for Europe on a milestone to be achieved between 2005 and 2010: to ensure representation of users and carers on committees and groups responsible for planning, delivering, reviewing and inspecting mental health activities.

Representation of service users on committees and groups responsible for mental health services

Representation was selected as an indicator of empowerment, since it can reflect respect and involvement. At best, representation means a voice in decision-making and, at worst, passive attendance without any power. It is hoped that representation would stand for the former level of involvement.

Definitions

In this chapter, service users, clients, patients and consumers are defined as the people receiving mental health care. These terms are used interchangeably in this report, as no one term is current in all settings and countries, and different groups of practitioners and people with mental disorders have traditionally used different terms. Their historical, cultural and personal meaning carry considerable significance (for example, patient implies to some people the passive receipt of health care), but this is beyond the scope of this report.

Carers or families are people who are living with, or informally looking after, people with mental health problems. This excludes the alternative of carer meaning employed mental health personnel.

Empowerment means giving increased responsibility and control to users and carers in planning services, treatment and care. The concept is based on a range of differing but not necessarily incompatible principles:

- moral and political concepts such as active citizenship;
- consumerism;
- concepts of product design and quality being fit for purpose and responsive; and
- enhancing control for therapeutic and humane reasons.

Table 10.1. Types of representation of service users in committees and groups that are common practice in groups of countries

Representation of service users in committees and groups responsible for mental health services	EU		EU15		New EU countries since 2004		Israel, Norway and Switzerland		South-eastern Europe		CIS		Total	
	No.	%	No.	%	No.	%	No.	%	No.	%	No.	%	No.	%
Planning														
Yes	16	59	12	80	4	33	1	33	3	43	0	0	20	48
No	9	33	2	13	7	58	0	0	4	57	5	100	18	43
Information not available	2	7	1	7	1	8	2	67	0	0	0	0	4	10
Implementation														
Yes	12	44	10	67	2	17	1	33	2	29	0	0	15	36
No	13	48	4	27	9	75	0	0	4	57	5	100	22	52
Information not available	2	7	1	7	1	8	2	67	1	14	0	0	5	12
Review														
Yes	15	56	11	73	4	33	1	33	1	14	0	0	17	40
No	10	37	3	20	7	58	0	0	5	71	4	80	19	45
Information not available	2	7	1	7	1	8	2	67	1	14	1	20	6	14

According to the survey responses, government directives cover the participation of service users in planning activities in 17 of the 42 countries (40%). Service users are represented on groups or committees responsible for planning mental health services in 20 of 42 countries (49%) (Tables 10.1 and 10.2). Users are involved in such committees in 12 of the EU15 countries (80%) and in 4 of the 12 countries that joined the EU after 2004 (33%). Austria, the Czech Republic, Denmark, Finland, Italy and the United Kingdom (Scotland) indicate that, although there are no directives, service users are represented on these committees in practice. No CIS country participating in the survey has policy requirements to ensure the representation of service users, and they are not involved in any of the activities of these committees in practice. This questionnaire does not enable the assessment of the consistency of the involvement of service users in the many national, regional and local planning groups or the impact and credibility of service users on committees. This is likely to vary not only between countries but also between places and meetings and to depend on the quality and interaction of both professionals and service users. Some countries recognize this, and several countries have given examples.

Some countries have well-defined requirements for the representation of service users on committees and groups responsible for planning mental health services.

- In Ireland, the recently adopted policy document *A vision for change* notes that change is also required from service users and carers, since much greater involvement and responsibility is envisaged for these groups. It also notes that service users must be at the centre of decision-making at the individual level in terms of the services available to them, in the strategic development of local services and in developing national policy.
- The Netherlands has a Law on Client Participation in Health Services, which requires every health service to institute a clients' council with strong advisory powers over the institution's policies, including the composition of the board.

Other countries have requirements to involve service users, but they are rather broad.

- In Italy, representation is suggested in the national policy (P.O. 1998–2000) but not with details regarding specific sectors.
- In Lithuania, the mental health strategy requires the involvement of service

Table 10.2. Representation of service users on committees and groups responsible for planning, implementing and reviewing mental health services required by government directives and common in practice in countries

	Government directives on the representation of service users on committees and groups responsible for mental health services:			Representation of service users on committees and groups responsible for mental health services:		
Country	Planning	Implementation	Review	Planning	Implementation	Review
Albania	Yes	Yes	Yes	Yes	No	No
Austria	No	No	No	Yes	No	No
Azerbaijan	No	No	No	No	No	No
Belgium	Yes	Yes	Yes	Yes	Yes	Yes
Bosnia and Herzegovina						
Federation of Bosnia and Herzegovina	Yes	Yes	Yes	Yes	Yes	No
Republika Srpska	Yes	Yes	Yes	Yes	Yes	No
Bulgaria	No	No	No	No	No	No
Croatia	No	Information not available	Information not available	No	Information not available	Information not available
Cyprus	No	No	No	No	No	No
Czech Republic	No	No	No	Yes	No	Yes
Denmark	No	No	No	Yes	Yes	Yes
Estonia	No	No	No	No	No	No
Finland	No	No	No	Yes	Yes	Yes
France	Yes	Yes	Yes	Yes	Yes	Yes
Georgia	No	No	No	No	No	No
Germany	Yes	Yes	Yes	Yes	Yes	Yes
Greece	No	No	No	No	No	No
Hungary	No	No	No	No	No	No
Ireland	Yes	Yes	Yes	Yes	Yes	Yes
Israel	Information not available	Information not available	Information not available	Information not available	Information not available	Information not available
Italy	No	No	No	Yes	Yes	Yes
Latvia	Yes	Yes	Yes	Yes	No	Yes
Lithuania	Yes	Yes	Yes	Yes	Yes	Yes
Luxembourg	Yes	Yes	Yes	Yes	Yes	Yes
Malta	No	No	No	No	No	No
Moldova	No	No	No	No	No	No
Montenegro	No	No	No	No	No	No
Netherlands	No	No	No	No	No	No
Norway	Yes	Yes	Yes	Yes	Yes	Yes
Poland	Yes	Yes	Information not available	No	No	No
Portugal	No	No	No	Information not available	Information not available	Information not available
Romania	No	No	No	No	No	No
Russian Federation	No	No	No	No	No	Information not available
Serbia	No	No	No	No	No	No
Slovakia	No	No	Yes	Information not available	Information not available	Information not available
Slovenia	Yes	Yes	Yes	Yes	Yes	Yes
Spain						
Castilla y León	Yes	No	No	Yes	No	No
Catalonia	Yes	Yes	Yes	Yes	No	Yes
Extremadura	Yes	Information not available	Yes	Yes	Information not available	Yes
Galicia	Information not available	No	No	Information not available	No	No
Murcia	No	No	No	No	No	No
Sweden	Yes	Yes	Yes	Yes	Yes	Yes
Switzerland	Yes	No	No	Information not available	Information not available	Information not available
The former Yugoslav Republic of Macedonia	Yes	Yes	Yes	Yes	Yes	Yes
Turkey	No	No	No	No	No	No
United Kingdom						
England and Wales	Yes	Yes	Yes	Yes	Yes	Yes
Scotland	No	No	No	Yes	Yes	Yes
Uzbekistan	No	No	No	No	No	No

Yes ■ No ■ Information not available

users. Details of how this policy will be implemented will be outlined in the upcoming action plan.

The type and level of involvement vary across regions in the same country (such as Italy and Sweden) and across countries.

- In Albania, service users are represented in the National Steering Committee for Mental Health.
- The Czech Republic service users' organization is an advisory group to the Ministry of Health.
- In France, the National Federation of Association of Users and Ex-Users of Psychiatry (Fnapsy) and the National Union of Friends and Families of People with Mental Illness (UNAFAM), the carers' organization, are represented in all the administrative commissions and meetings relating to mental health conducted by the Minister for Health.
- In Italy, service users' associations are still relatively rare but are involved where they exist.
- In Latvia, service users have an advisory function for the "Special Regular Work Body" in the Ministry of Health.
- In the Netherlands, service users and carers are consulted in the design of care programmes and treatment guidelines. Individual institutions consult organizations of service users on specific themes. It is not common practice to have service users or carers represented on planning, implementation or review commissions.
- In Georgia, two representatives from the organization of service users and carers are members of the Mental Health Policy Development Council in the Ministry. This involvement is formal.
- However, in Bulgaria, where the board of trustees of hospitals is the only body with representation of service users, the Health Facilities Act stipulates that a board of trustees will not be established for mental health hospitals.

Fewer countries (15 of 42) indicate that service users are represented on committees and groups responsible for implementing policy on mental health services (Table 10.2). Service users' involvement in monitoring the implementation of services is most frequent in the EU15 countries (10 of 15) and least in CIS countries. None of the CIS countries report that government directives formally require such representation or that this is common practice.

Denmark, Finland, Italy and the United Kingdom (Scotland) indicate that, although there are no formal requirements, service users are nevertheless involved in committees and groups responsible for implementing mental health services. Similar to other policy areas, several countries report that existing formal requirements are not translated into practice (Albania, Latvia, Poland and Spain (Catalonia)). This is probably common.

Finally, service users are reported to be represented on committees and groups responsible for reviewing mental health services in 17 of 42 countries. In five countries (the Czech Republic, Denmark, Finland, Italy and the United Kingdom (Scotland)), service users are represented on these committees by choice rather than in response to government directives. In contrast, in some countries in which policy requires that service users be represented, they are not involved in such committees in practice (in Albania, Bosnia and Herzegovina (Federation of Bosnia and Herzegovina and Republika Srpska) or information is not available on their actual involvement (Slovakia). Such countries as Sweden and Switzerland note local variation within the country in the involvement of service users in such committees.

Representation of service users on committees and groups responsible for anti-stigma, mental disorder prevention and mental health promotion activities

The rationale for having service users on committees addressing anti-stigma activities is that they have been subject to the stigma and resulting discrimination and can therefore advise based on the strength of personal experiences. More complex is the case for involvement in activities for preventing

Table. 10.3. Representation of service users on committees and groups responsible for planning, implementing and reviewing anti-stigma, mental disorder prevention and mental health promotion activities required by government directives and common in practice in countries

Country	Government directives on the representation of service users on committees and groups responsible for anti-stigma, mental disorder prevention and mental health promotion activities:			Representation of service users on committees and groups responsible for anti-stigma, mental disorder prevention and mental health promotion activities:		
	Planning	Implementation	Review	Planning	Implementation	Review
Albania	Yes	Yes	Yes	Yes	No	No
Austria	No	No	No	Yes	No	No
Azerbaijan	No	No	No	No	No	No
Belgium	Yes	Yes	Yes	Yes	Yes	Yes
Bosnia and Herzegovina						
Federation of Bosnia and Herzegovina	Yes	Yes	Yes	Yes	Information not available	No
Republika Srpska	Yes	Yes	Yes	Yes	Yes	No
Bulgaria	No	No	No	No	No	No
Croatia	No	Yes	Yes	No	Yes	Yes
Cyprus	No	No	No	No	No	No
Czech Republic	No	No	No	Information not available	No	Information not available
Denmark	No	No	No	Yes	Yes	Yes
Estonia	No	No	No	No	No	No
Finland	No	No	No	Yes	Yes	Yes
France	Information not available	Information not available	Information not available	Information not available	Information not available	Information not available
Georgia	No	No	No	Yes	No	No
Germany	Yes	Yes	Yes	Yes	Yes	No
Greece	No	No	No	No	No	No
Hungary	No	No	No	No	No	No
Ireland	Yes	Yes	Yes	Information not available	Information not available	Information not available
Israel	Information not available	Information not available	Information not available	Information not available	Information not available	Information not available
Italy	No	No	No	Yes	Yes	Yes
Latvia	No	No	No	Yes	No	Yes
Lithuania	Yes	Yes	Yes	Yes	Yes	Yes
Luxembourg	Information not available	Information not available	Information not available	Information not available	Information not available	Information not available
Malta	No	No	No	No	No	No
Moldova	No	No	No	No	No	No
Montenegro	No	No	No	No	No	No
Netherlands	No	No	No	No	No	No
Norway	Yes	Yes	Yes	Yes	Yes	Yes
Poland	Yes	Yes	Information not available	Yes	Yes	No
Portugal	No	No	No	Information not available	Information not available	Information not available
Romania	No	No	No	No	No	No
Russian Federation	No	No	No	No	No	Yes
Serbia	No	Yes	Yes	No	No	No
Slovakia	No	No	Information not available	Information not available	Information not available	Information not available
Slovenia	Yes	Yes	Yes	Yes	Yes	Yes
Spain						
Castilla y León	Yes	No	No	Yes	No	No
Catalonia	Yes	Yes	Yes	Yes	No	Yes
Extremadura	Yes	Yes	Yes	Yes	Yes	Yes
Galicia	Yes	No	No	Yes	No	No
Murcia	No	No	No	No	No	No
Sweden	Yes	Yes	Yes	Information not available	Information not available	Information not available
Switzerland	Information not available	Information not available	Information not available	Information not available	Information not available	Information not available
The former Yugoslav Republic of Macedonia	Yes	Yes	Yes	Yes	Yes	Yes
Turkey	No	No	No	No	No	No
United Kingdom						
England and Wales	Yes	Yes	Yes	Yes	Yes	Yes
Scotland	No	No	No	Information not available	Information not available	Information not available
Uzbekistan	No	No	No	No	No	No

Yes No Information not available

Table 10.4. Types of representation of families or carers in committees and groups that are common practice in groups of countries

Representation of families or carers in committees and groups responsible for mental health services	EU		EU15		New EU countries since 2004		Israel, Norway and Switzerland		South-eastern Europe		CIS		Total	
	No.	%	No.	%	No.	%	No.	%	No.	%	No.	%	No.	%
Planning														
Yes	16	59	12	80	4	33	1	33	3	43	0	0	20	48
No	9	33	1	7	8	67	0	0	4	57	4	80	17	40
Information not available	2	7	2	13	0	0	2	67	0	0	1	20	5	12
Implementation														
Yes	14	52	11	73	3	25	1	33	3	43	0	0	18	43
No	11	41	2	13	9	75	0	0	3	43	4	80	18	43
Information not available	2	7	2	13	0	0	2	67	1	14	1	20	6	14
Review														
Yes	15	56	11	73	4	33	1	33	2	29	1	20	19	45
No	10	37	2	13	8	67	0	0	4	57	4	80	18	43
Information not available	2	7	2	13	0	0	2	67	1	14	0	0	5	12

mental disorders and promoting mental health, since the target groups for mental disorder prevention are people at risk and, for mental health promotion, the general public. Representatives need to be selected based on background and expertise relevant to the planned activities. The meaning of service user needs to be interpreted broadly in this section, referring to members of the target groups with some relevant experience and credibility.

Slightly fewer countries (17 of 42) indicate that users are represented on committees and groups responsible for planning anti-stigma, mental disorder prevention and mental health promotion activities (Table 10.3) compared with planning mental health services (20 of 42 countries). In Austria, Denmark, Finland, Italy, Georgia (the only CIS country to report such involvement) and Latvia, service users are usually involved in anti-stigma activities, even though there are no specific policy requirements for this. Ireland and Sweden have adopted government directives requiring the representation of service users on such committees, but information is not available on whether this practice is common or not.

Six of the EU15 countries and 3 of the 12 countries joining the EU since 2004 require the involvement of service users on committees responsible for implementing anti-stigma, mental disorder prevention and mental health promotion activities. Only about a third of the countries report that service users are indeed represented on committees or groups responsible for implementing and reviewing anti-stigma, mental disorder prevention and mental health promotion activities.

Denmark, Finland and Italy report that no government directives support service users' involvement in committees implementing activities, but service users are often represented in practice. Additionally, Latvia and the Russian Federation indicate that service users are active in committees dealing with reviewing anti-stigma, mental disorder prevention and mental health promotion activities, although government directives do not specifically require this.

Representation of families or carers on committees and groups responsible for mental health services

The involvement of carers in planning mental health services is similar to that of service users: 18 of 42 countries have adopted government directives requiring their representation

Table 10.5. Representation of carers on committees and groups responsible for planning, implementing and reviewing mental health services required by government directives and common in practice in countries

Country	Government directives on the representation of carers on committees and groups responsible for mental health services:			Representation of carers on committees and groups responsible for mental health services:		
	Planning	Implementation	Review	Planning	Implementation	Review
Albania	Yes	Yes	Yes	Yes	No	No
Austria	No	No	No	Yes	No	No
Azerbaijan	No	No	No	No	No	No
Belgium	Yes	Yes	Yes	Yes	Yes	Yes
Bosnia and Herzegovina						
Federation of Bosnia and Herzegovina	Yes	Yes	No	No	No	No
Republika Srpska	Yes	Yes	Yes	Information not available	Yes	No
Bulgaria	No	No	No	No	No	No
Croatia	No	Information not available	Information not available	No	Information not available	Information not available
Cyprus	No	No	No	No	No	No
Czech Republic	No	No	No	Yes	No	Yes
Denmark	No	No	No	Yes	Yes	Yes
Estonia	No	No	No	No	No	No
Finland	No	No	No	Yes	Yes	Yes
France	Yes	Yes	Yes	Yes	Yes	Yes
Georgia	Information not available	No	No	No	No	No
Germany	Yes	Yes	Yes	Yes	Yes	Yes
Greece	No	No	No	No	No	No
Hungary	No	No	No	No	No	No
Ireland	Yes	Yes	Yes	Yes	Yes	Yes
Israel	Information not available	Information not available	Information not available	Information not available	Information not available	Information not available
Italy	No	No	No	Yes	Yes	Yes
Latvia	No	No	No	Yes	Yes	Yes
Lithuania	Yes	Yes	Yes	Yes	Yes	Yes
Luxembourg	Yes	Yes	Yes	Yes	Yes	Yes
Malta	No	No	No	No	No	No
Moldova	Information not available	Information not available	Information not available	No	No	No
Montenegro	No	No	No	No	No	No
Netherlands	No	No	No	Information not available	Information not available	Information not available
Norway	Yes	Yes	Yes	Yes	Yes	Yes
Poland	Information not available	Information not available	Information not available	No	No	No
Portugal	Yes	No	No	Information not available	Information not available	Information not available
Romania	No	No	No	No	No	No
Russian Federation	No	No	No	Information not available	Information not available	Yes
Serbia	No	No	No	No	No	No
Slovakia	Yes	Yes	Yes	No	No	No
Slovenia	Yes	Yes	Yes	Yes	Yes	Yes
Spain						
Castilla y León	Yes	Yes	No	Yes	Yes	Information not available
Catalonia	Yes	Yes	Yes	Yes	No	Yes
Extremadura	Yes	Information not available	Yes	Yes	Information not available	Yes
Galicia	Information not available	No	No	Information not available	No	No
Murcia	No	No	No	No	No	No
Sweden	Yes	Yes	Yes	Yes	Yes	Yes
Switzerland	Yes	No	No	Information not available	Information not available	Information not available
The former Yugoslav Republic of Macedonia	Yes	Yes	Yes	Yes	Yes	Yes
Turkey	Yes	Yes	Yes	Yes	Yes	Yes
United Kingdom						
England and Wales	Yes	Yes	Yes	Yes	Yes	Yes
Scotland	No	No	No	Yes	Yes	Yes
Uzbekistan	No	No	No	No	No	No

Yes · No · Information not available

on groups and committees, and 20 of 42 countries report that this is common practice (Table 10.4).

In Austria, the Czech Republic, Denmark, Finland, Italy, Latvia and the United Kingdom (Scotland), carers participate in planning activities despite the absence of directives (Table 10.5). In some countries where carers' participation is required, they are either not involved in practice (Bosnia and Herzegovina (Federation of Bosnia and Herzegovina) and Slovakia) or information about involvement is not available (Bosnia and Herzegovina (Republika Srpska), Portugal and Switzerland).

Examples of carers' involvement in planning mental health services are identical to the examples of the involvement of service users. In most countries, service users and carers are probably regularly invited to the same meetings. Although this is positive in principle, it would be interesting to have examples of how the opinions of these groups, which can represent very different interests in some circumstances, are distinguished and the influence of each type of opinion.

Carers' role in implementing and reviewing mental health services again reflects user representation closely, both for policy requirements and practice. Denmark, Finland, Italy, Latvia and the United Kingdom (Scotland) involve carers in practice in implementing services, but without written policies, and 14 of 42 countries combine policy and good practice. Altogether, 18 of 42 countries indicate carers' representatives commonly participate in practice in committees and groups responsible for monitoring mental health services. In Turkey, service users are not involved in either of these types of committees, but carers are reported to be involved in all of them.

Representation of families or carers on committees and groups responsible for anti-stigma, mental disorder prevention and mental health promotion activities

Representatives of carers, as was the case for users, need to be selected based on relevance. Their relevance is high for anti-stigma activities but depends on the type of activity and target group for promoting mental health and preventing mental disorders.

Carers are more likely to be represented on committees and groups that implement (14 of 42 countries) rather than on those that monitor or review the implementation of anti-stigma, mental disorder prevention and mental health promotion activities (11 of 42 countries).

None of the CIS countries report the involvement of service users on these committees, but two (Georgia and the Russian Federation) indicate that carers are represented.

In Austria, Denmark, Finland, Italy and the Russian Federation, families and carers are represented on committees and groups responsible for planning, implementing and reviewing anti-stigma, mental disorder prevention and mental health promotion activities, although there are no directives. In Austria and Georgia, they are represented only on planning committees.

Government support for organizations of service users and carers

Governments need to support organizations of service users and carers both financially and by providing infrastructure to ensure the availability of the expertise of service users and carers for planning, implementing and reviewing activities. This can be delivered either by central funding or by directives and earmarked money, aiming to stimulate local developments.

Table 10.6. Representation of carers on committees and groups responsible for planning, implementing and reviewing anti-stigma, mental disorder prevention and mental health promotion activities required by government directives and common in practice in countries

Country	Government directives on the representation of carers on committees and groups responsible for anti-stigma, mental disorder prevention and mental health promotion activities:			Representation of carers on committees and groups responsible for anti-stigma, mental disorder prevention and mental health promotion activities:		
	Planning	Implementation	Review	Planning	Implementation	Review
Albania	Yes	Yes	Yes	Yes	No	No
Austria	No	No	No	Yes	No	No
Azerbaijan	No	No	No	No	No	No
Belgium	Yes	Yes	Yes	Yes	Yes	Yes
Bosnia and Herzegovina						
Federation of Bosnia and Herzegovina	Yes	Yes	No	No	No	No
Republika Srpska	Yes	Yes	Yes	Yes	Yes	No
Bulgaria	No	No	No	No	No	No
Croatia	No	Yes	Yes	No	Yes	Yes
Cyprus	No	No	No	No	No	No
Czech Republic	No	No	No	Information not available	No	Information not available
Denmark	No	No	No	Yes	Yes	Yes
Estonia	No	No	No	No	No	No
Finland	No	No	No	Yes	Yes	Yes
France	Information not available	Information not available	Information not available	Information not available	Information not available	Information not available
Georgia	No	No	No	Yes	No	No
Germany	Yes	Yes	Yes	Yes	Yes	No
Greece	No	No	No	No	No	No
Hungary	No	No	No	No	No	No
Ireland	Yes	Yes	Yes	Information not available	Information not available	Information not available
Israel	Information not available	Information not available	Information not available	Information not available	Information not available	Information not available
Italy	No	No	No	Yes	Yes	Yes
Latvia	No	No	No	No	No	No
Lithuania	Yes	Yes	Yes	Yes	Yes	Yes
Luxembourg	Information not available	Information not available	Information not available	Information not available	Information not available	Information not available
Malta	No	No	No	No	No	No
Moldova	Information not available	Information not available	Information not available	No	No	No
Montenegro	No	No	No	No	No	No
Netherlands	No	No	No	Information not available	Information not available	Information not available
Norway	Yes	Yes	Yes	Yes	Yes	Yes
Poland	Information not available	Information not available	Information not available	No	No	No
Portugal	Yes	No	No	Information not available	Information not available	Information not available
Romania	No	No	No	No	No	No
Russian Federation	No	No	No	Yes	Yes	Yes
Serbia	No	Yes	Yes	No	No	No
Slovakia	Information not available	Information not available	Information not available	No	No	No
Slovenia	Yes	Yes	Yes	Yes	Yes	Yes
Spain						
Castilla y León	Yes	Yes	No	Yes	Yes	Information not available
Catalonia	Yes	Yes	Yes	Yes	No	Yes
Extremadura	Yes	Yes	Yes	Yes	Yes	Yes
Galicia	Yes	No	No	Yes	No	No
Murcia	No	No	No	No	No	No
Sweden	Information not available	Information not available	Information not available	Information not available	Information not available	Information not available
Switzerland	Information not available	Information not available	Information not available	Information not available	Information not available	Information not available
The former Yugoslav Republic of Macedonia	Yes	Yes	Yes	Yes	Yes	Information not available
Turkey	Information not available	Information not available	Information not available	Information not available	Information not available	Information not available
United Kingdom						
England and Wales	Yes	Yes	Yes	Yes	Yes	Yes
Scotland	No	No	No	Information not available	Information not available	Information not available
Uzbekistan	No	No	No	No	No	No

Yes ■ No ■ Information not available

Table 10.7. Systematic government funding for establishing and operating associations of service users or consumers and associations of family members or carers in groups of countries

Associations with government funding	EU		EU15		New EU countries since 2004		Israel, Norway and Switzerland		South-eastern Europe		CIS		Total	
	No.	%	No.	%	No.	%	No.	%	No.	%	No.	%	No.	%
Service users or consumers														
Yes	13	48	11	73	2	17	2	67	1	14	0	0	16	38
No	13	48	3	20	10	83	0	0	6	86	5	100	24	57
Information not available	1	4	1	7	0	0	1	33	0	0	0	0	2	5
Family members or carers														
Yes	12	44	10	67	2	17	2	67	1	14	0	0	15	36
No	14	52	4	27	10	83	0	0	6	86	5	100	25	60
Information not available	1	4	1	7	0	0	1	33	0	0	0	0	2	5

Only 2 of the 12 countries that have joined the EU since 2004 (Estonia and Slovenia), 1 of the 7 countries in south-eastern Europe and none of the CIS countries report that governments fund the establishment and operation of associations of service users or consumers or associations of family members or carers (Table 10.7).

Such funding is made available for associations of service users or consumers in most of the EU15 countries. The exceptions are Finland, Greece and Italy, which do not formally support these associations. However, local government and charities provide considerable funding for associations in Finland.

Similarly, associations of family members and carers also receive national funding in all but four EU15 countries (Finland, Greece, Italy and Sweden), but for Finland the carers' support is identical to the service users' funding. Information about government support for organizations of service users or carers is not available for Portugal.

Of the countries indicating that government funds these associations, the level of funding differs substantially.

- In Bosnia and Herzegovina (Federation of Bosnia and Herzegovina) with two associations of service users, funds are made available in many of the regions but not every year. In Tuzla, the local government allocates small amounts yearly (€10 000 to €15 000 in 2007).
- In Bulgaria, local governments in some regions provide support to nongovernmental organizations and collaborate to create a local mental health policy.
- In the Russian Federation, governments do not fund activities; charities fund them or they are carried out by volunteers.
- In Germany, support is low. Examples of government funding include:
  - family self-help (Federal Association of Relatives of Mentally Ill People (BApK));
  - Federal Organization of (ex-)Users and Survivors of Psychiatry in Germany (BPE);
  - promotion of self-help associations in the individual Länder; and
  - the governments of the Länder fund consumer organizations.

Between 16 and 19 countries report that governments provide targeted funding for associations of service users and carers active in:

- providing community-based services involving service users;
- developing the caring and coping skills and competencies of families and carers;
- developing and implementing mental health promotion and mental disorder prevention initiatives for service users and carers; and
- advocacy and legal representation of the rights of service users (Table 10.8).

Table 10.8. Initiatives for service users and carers in countries

Country	Providing community-based services involving users – government provides financial support	Developing the caring and coping skills and competencies of families and carers – government provides financial support	Developing and implementing mental health promotion and prevention initiatives for service users and carers – government provides financial support	Advocacy and empowerment of service users' rights – government provides financial support
Albania	No	No	No	No
Austria	Information not available	Information not available	Information not available	Information not available
Azerbaijan	No	No	No	No
Belgium	Information not available	Yes	Information not available	Yes
Bosnia and Herzegovina				
Federation of Bosnia and Herzegovina	No	Yes	Yes	Yes
Republika Srpska	Yes	Yes	Yes	Yes
Bulgaria	No	No	No	No
Croatia	Yes	Yes	Yes	Yes
Cyprus	Yes	No	No	No
Czech Republic	No	No	No	No
Denmark	Information not available	Yes	Yes	Yes
Estonia	Yes	Yes	Yes	Yes
Finland	No	No	No	No
France	Yes	Yes	No	Yes
Georgia	No	No	No	No
Germany	Yes	Yes	Yes	Yes
Greece	Yes	No	Yes	No
Hungary	Yes	No	No	No
Ireland	Yes	Yes	Yes	Yes
Israel	Information not available	Information not available	Information not available	Information not available
Italy	No	No	No	No
Latvia	No	No	No	No
Lithuania	Yes	Yes	Yes	Yes
Luxembourg	Yes	Yes	Yes	Yes
Malta	Yes	No	No	No
Moldova	No	No	No	No
Montenegro	No	No	No	No
Netherlands	Information not available	Yes	Yes	Yes
Norway	Yes	Yes	Yes	Yes
Poland	Yes	No	Information not available	No
Portugal	No	No	No	No
Romania	No	No	No	No
Russian Federation	No	No	Yes	No
Serbia	No	No	Information not available	Yes
Slovakia	No	No	No	No
Slovenia	Yes	No	Yes	Yes
Spain				
Castilla y León	Yes	Yes	Yes	Yes
Catalonia	Yes	Yes	Yes	Yes
Extremadura	Yes	Yes	Yes	Information not available
Galicia	Yes	Yes	Yes	Yes
Murcia	Yes	Yes	Yes	Yes
Sweden	Yes	Yes	Yes	Yes
Switzerland	Yes	Yes	No	Yes
The former Yugoslav Republic of Macedonia	No	No	No	No
Turkey	No	No	No	No
United Kingdom				
England and Wales	Yes	Yes	Yes	Yes
Scotland	Yes	Yes	Yes	Yes
Uzbekistan	No	No	No	No

Yes No Information not available

Governments in the EU15 countries are very active in all these areas. This survey cannot identify the level and range of funding, which probably differs considerably. For example, in some countries, funding can comprise regular earmarked grants available for initiatives in these areas. Other countries rely on small-scale initiatives from nongovernmental organizations they fund.

Main activities initiated and developed since 2005 related to empowering mental health service users and carers

Activities aimed at empowering service users and carers have been initiated and developed in many countries. The following are examples.

Establishment of organizations of service users

- Italy: establishment of the National Council of Associations (Consulta delle associazioni, http://www.ministerosalute.it/saluteMentale/paginaSempliceSaluteMentale.jsp?id=391&menu=consulta).

Representation on boards and committees

- Albania: involvement of representatives of associations of service users and carers on the National Steering Committee for Mental Health.
- Austria: service users and carers are represented on the Advisory Board for Mental Health at the Austrian Federal Ministry of Health.
- Czech Republic: service users participate in an advisory group of the Ministry of Health.
- Ireland: the Health Service Executive established an interim National Service User Executive in January 2007. Service users are part of the National Mental Health Expert Advisory Group. Service users are invited to take part in interview boards for staff selection. Additional investment has been made in advocacy services through voluntary organizations. Peer advocacy is available in all acute admission sites and many community service sites.

Support for organizations of service users

- Bosnia and Herzegovina (Federation of Bosnia and Herzegovina): the Ministry of Health grants some funds to associations of service users and family members. This practice became regular after the WHO European Ministerial Conference on Mental Health.
- In Finland, the municipalities fund nongovernmental organizations and not the government. On a national level, the main source of funding is Finland's Slot Machine Association.
- Germany: the health insurance funds promote the further development of patient and consumer counselling. The establishment of an association for independent patient counselling in Germany has given rise to a national network of independent counselling services (22 local counselling offices, 4 services extending beyond local regions and a unified national telephone counselling hotline) since January 2007.
- Norway: the perspective of service users has been a very strong focus in Norway during the past decade. An action plan for including service users was published in 2006.

Countries with no developments since 2005 are Azerbaijan, Bulgaria, Croatia, Greece, Malta, Montenegro, Portugal, Romania, Slovakia, Switzerland and Uzbekistan. Information is not available for Belgium, Poland and Turkey.

Discussion

This chapter identified the extent to which service users and carers are recognized as partners in the decision-making process in planning, implementing and monitoring mental health services and in mental health promotion, mental disorder prevention and anti-stigma activities in European countries.

Associations of service users and consumers and of family members and carers are entitled to be members of such committees and groups in many countries. The findings need to be interpreted in the light of the different cultures and economies of the countries, some relying more strongly on explicit policy statements and directives than others, some stimulating the development of civil society more than others and some having more money to allocate to groups.

Several conclusions emerge.

1. There is a strong correlation between trends in mental health expenditure, trends in the development of community mental health services and the involvement of users and carers. These are thus strongest among the EU15 countries. In many countries in the eastern part of the WHO European Region where the institutional model of care still dominates, user and carer movements are in a developmental stage. A survey of this kind cannot provide insight into the characteristics of organizations in different parts of the Region, but many nongovernmental organizations in western Europe are large and sophisticated agencies with high levels of funding. In some CIS countries, service user groups are small scale and often initiated and led by highly committed psychiatrists, with minimal funding that may have been obtained from foreign donors. Although it is questionable whether such groups are proper service user groups, there have been examples where such small beginnings lead to powerful developments.
2. It is not surprising that various representative rights are strongly correlated: if service users and carers are involved in planning, they are likely to be involved in implementation and monitoring. This reflects the culture of the country and the stage of development of mental health services. Moreover, the respective rights of service users and carers are very similar, both in directives or regulation and in practice. This applies to country groups and to individual countries. At one level this is not a surprise, since service users and carers are often perceived as equally worthy, and joint representation seems to achieve a fair balance. However, it would be of concern if service users and carers and their representative groups were seen as being interchangeable or being included as a gesture rather than standing for a unique perspective. A more sophisticated form of representation may need to be developed that offers the respective groups rights and involvement based on their needs but also based on their unique expertise.
3. Although representation on formal committees is often a formality currently in some countries, a high number of countries reporting policies that support representation is a sign of increasing awareness of the acceptance in principle that the beneficiaries of the services and their families and carers should have a say in their treatment and care. However, it is also clear that strong representation can occur in the absence of regulation, and regulation alone is not sufficient. A culture of empowerment and mutual respect may be more important than legislation in practice.
4. It can be underestimated how demanding and stressful representation can be for people who recently were subjected to treatment, possibly compulsory, from the same authorities with whom they are now sitting at the table on a presumed equal basis. It is hardly surprising that service users and carers can be perceived as silent without any significant contribution to make. Support and training is necessary and should be a component of user empowerment if it is to be taken seriously. At the very least, more than a single representative should be invited.

The data in this chapter clearly raise many questions, particularly qualitative in nature. It would be of particular interest to determine the influence of groups of service users and carers on policy and practice, both at the national and local levels, and how this is related to other political, social, cultural and economic factors. It is hopeful that the importance and rights of groups of service users and carers are recognized in so many countries, but it is also clear that further progress can be made, and this deserves to be monitored over the next few years.

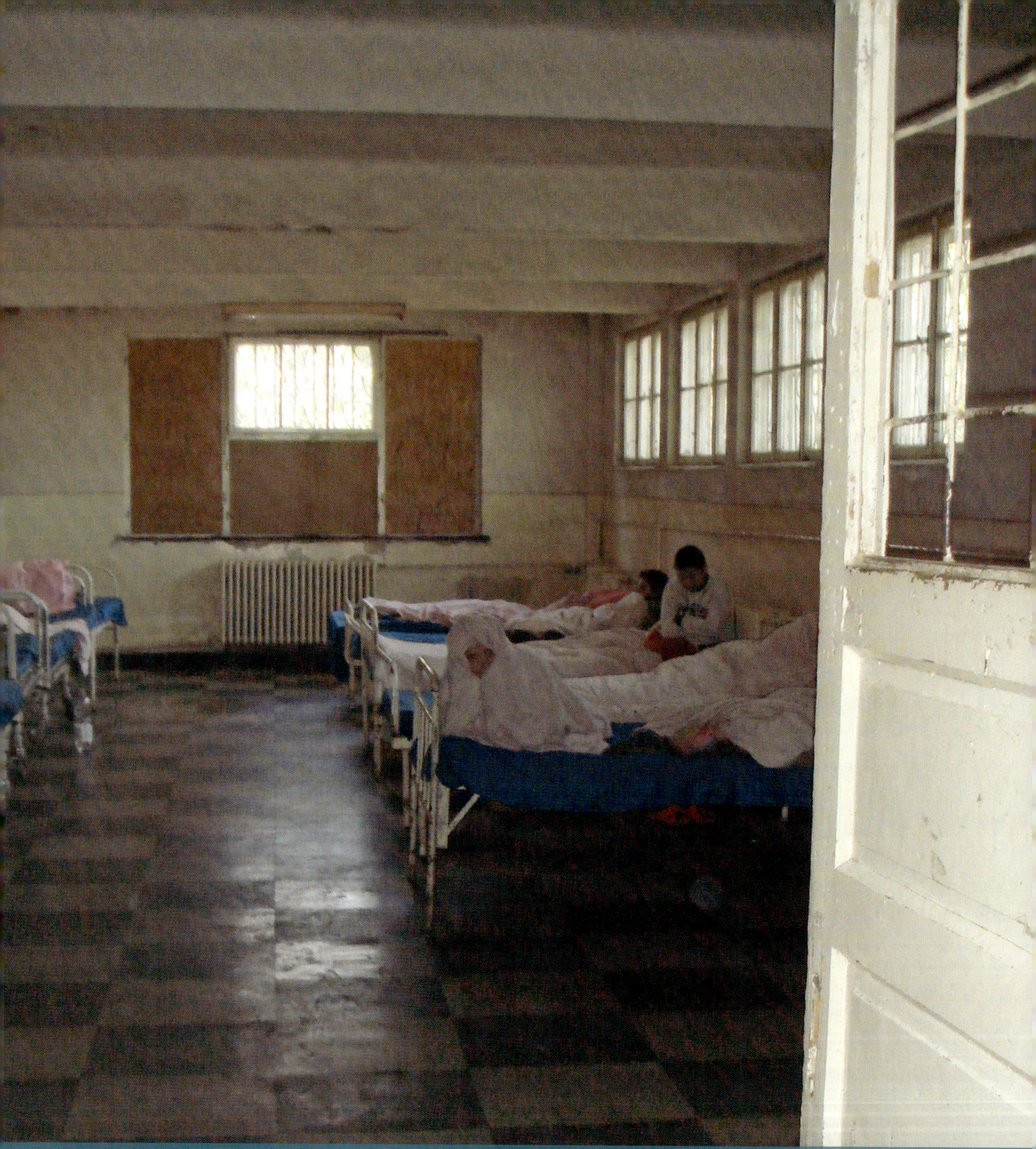

PHOTO © IONELA PETREA

“Human rights protection is a central issue in the care of people with mental health problems, who are vulnerable and exposed to neglect and abuse”

11. Human rights and mental health

People with mental health problems are among the most vulnerable people in society and can find themselves in circumstances where they require protection. This chapter focuses on the mental health service element of protecting human rights.

Human rights is a key consideration for the development and quality of mental health interventions and services. Many human right conventions refer either directly or indirectly to the rights of people with mental health problems and the duty of the state and service providers[1, 2]. Conventions relate to discrimination, quality of access and care, protection against neglect and abuse and safeguards in the case of treatment or care without consent by the person being treated.

Protecting the human rights of people with mental health problems remains a major challenge in the WHO European Region, emphasized by the many countries in which treatment and care for mental disorders is provided mainly in large institutions, either psychiatric hospitals or social care institutions. The Mental Health Declaration for Europe sets a milestone for all Member States to "end inhumane and degrading treatment and care and enact human rights and mental health legislation to comply with the standards of United Nations conventions and international legislation".

Definitions

Review bodies are agencies or group of people responsible for monitoring, reviewing, inspecting or checking the functions, operations or conditions of health services.

Restraint means the limitation or restriction of movement due to the application of a mechanical device or chemical means.

Involuntary admission refers to admission to mental health facilities that occurs without the voluntary consent of the individual. Involuntary admission is typically permitted when a person with a mental disorder is likely to cause self-harm or harm to others or suffer deterioration in condition if treatment is not given. Involuntary admission is typically governed by mental health legislation.

Seclusion is the state of being locked away on one's own for a period of time.

Mechanisms in place to monitor and review the human rights protection of users of mental health services

A key part of protecting human rights is monitoring and reviewing the conditions and practices in care institutions. Table 11.1 shows the functions of national and/or regional review bodies assessing the human rights protection of users in mental health services. Countries were asked to indicate whether national-level and/or regional-level review bodies have the following functions:

- regularly inspecting mental health facilities;
- reviewing involuntary admission and discharge procedures;
- reviewing processes of investigating complaints;
- reviewing the restriction of liberty;
- reviewing restraints; and
- imposing sanctions (such as withdrawing accreditation, imposing penalties or closing facilities that persistently violate human rights).

Most of the 42 countries have national and/or regional review bodies assessing the human rights protection of the users of mental health services. The EU15 countries especially have the most comprehensive monitoring mechanisms in place. Only four countries (Azerbaijan, Latvia, Lithuania and Turkey) indicate that national- or regional-level review bodies perform none of these functions.

1 *WHO resource book on mental health, human rights and legislation.* Geneva, World Health Organization, 2005 (http://www.who.int/mental_health/policy/legislation/policy/en, accessed 8 May 2008).

2 *Mental health legislation and human rights* (Mental health policy and service guidance package). Geneva, World Health Organization, 2003 (http://www.who.int/mental_health/resources/en/Legislation.pdf, accessed 8 May 2008).

Table 11.1. Functions of national and/or regional review bodies assessing the human rights protection of the users of mental health services in countries

Country	Performing regular inspection in mental health facilities	Reviewing involuntary admission and discharge procedures	Reviewing complaints investigation processes	Reviewing restriction of liberties	Reviewing restraint	Imposing sanctions (such as withdrawing accreditation, imposing penalties or closing facilities that persistently violate human rights)
Albania	Yes	Yes	No	No	No	No
Austria	Yes	Yes	Yes	Yes	Yes	No
Azerbaijan	No	No	No	No	No	No
Belgium	Yes	Yes	Yes	Yes	Yes	Yes
Bosnia and Herzegovina						
Federation of Bosnia and Herzegovina	Yes	Yes	Yes	Yes	Yes	Yes
Republika Srpska	Yes	Yes	Yes	Yes	Yes	Yes
Bulgaria	Yes	Yes	No	Yes	Yes	No
Croatia	Yes	Yes	Yes	Yes	Yes	Yes
Cyprus	Yes	Yes	Yes	Yes	Yes	No
Czech Republic	Yes	Yes	Yes	Yes	Yes	Yes
Denmark	Yes	Yes	Yes	Yes	Yes	Yes
Estonia	Yes	Yes	Yes	Yes	Yes	Yes
Finland	Yes	Yes	Yes	Yes	Yes	Yes
France	Yes	Yes	Yes	Yes	Yes	Yes
Georgia	Yes	Yes	Yes	Yes	Yes	No
Germany	Yes	Yes	Yes	Yes	Yes	Yes
Greece	Yes	Yes	Yes	Information not available	Yes	No
Hungary	No	Yes	Yes	Information not available	Yes	Information not available
Ireland	Yes	Yes	Yes	Yes	Yes	Yes
Israel	Information not available	Information not available	Information not available	Information not available	Information not available	Information not available
Italy	Yes	Yes	Yes	Yes	Yes	Yes
Latvia	No	No	No	No	No	No
Lithuania	No	No	No	No	No	No
Luxembourg	Yes	Yes	Yes	Yes	Yes	Yes
Malta	No	No	Yes	No	No	No
Moldova	Information not available	Information not available	Information not available	Information not available	Information not available	Information not available
Montenegro	Information not available	Information not available	Information not available	Information not available	Information not available	Information not available
Netherlands	Yes	Yes	Yes	Yes	Yes	Yes
Norway	Yes	Yes	Yes	Yes	Yes	Yes
Poland	Yes	Yes	Yes	Yes	Yes	No
Portugal	No	Yes	Yes	No	No	Information not available
Romania	Yes	Yes	Yes	Yes	Yes	Yes
Russian Federation	No	Yes	Yes	Yes	No	No
Serbia	Yes	Yes	Yes	Yes	Yes	No
Slovakia	Yes	Yes	Information not available	Yes	Information not available	Information not available
Slovenia	Yes	Yes	Yes	Yes	Yes	No
Spain						
Castilla y León	Yes	Yes	Yes	Yes	Yes	Yes
Catalonia	No	Yes	Yes	Yes	Yes	Yes
Extremadura	Information not available	Yes	Yes	Yes	Information not available	Yes
Galicia	No	No	Yes	No	No	No
Murcia	Information not available	Yes	Yes	Yes	Information not available	Information not available
Sweden	Yes	Yes	Yes	Yes	Yes	Yes
Switzerland	No	Yes	No	Yes	Yes	Yes
The former Yugoslav Republic of Macedonia	Yes	Yes	Yes	Yes	Yes	Yes
Turkey	No	No	No	No	No	No
United Kingdom						
England and Wales	Yes	Yes	Yes	Yes	Yes	Yes
Scotland	No	Yes	Yes	Yes	Yes	No
Uzbekistan	Yes	Yes	Yes	Yes	Yes	Yes

Yes No Information not available

Countries vary in the functions covered by review bodies. The most frequent function is the reviewing of involuntary admission and discharge procedures undertaken in 34 of 42 countries. Review bodies review complaint investigation procedures in 31 of 42 countries.

The function least frequently implemented in the participating countries is imposing sanctions, which is within the remit of review bodies in 21 of 42 countries. In many of the other countries, it may be assumed that review bodies will submit recommendations to other parties such as ministries, which will have the power to act.

Some countries have well-established mechanisms for monitoring the protection of human rights of people with mental health problems.

- In Italy, ad hoc national commissions appointed by the Parliament perform some tasks for specific problems, as do regional councils on mental health. Other responsibilities are part of the tasks of local bioethics committees. Finally, a national body called the Tribunal for Patients' Rights has a role to play.
- In the United Kingdom (England and Wales), the Mental Health Act Commission (soon to be merged with the Healthcare Commission and the Commission for Social Care Inspection to form the Care Quality Commission) regularly visits hospitals and closely monitors the patterns of involuntary admissions, including distribution by sex and ethnicity. It publishes a detailed annual report highlighting areas of concern. The Healthcare Commission performs annual ratings of the quality of hospital care, including the environment and staff and patient evaluations.

In other countries, arms-length groups undertake the functions of review bodies, either appointed by governments or at the initiative of nongovernmental organizations.

- In Albania, the review bodies are mainly teams of experts sent by the Ministry of Health to review the mental health facilities.
- In Bulgaria, the only organization which monitors psychiatric establishments in practice is a nongovernmental organization that has an agreement with the Ministry of Health for regular monitoring – the Bulgarian Helsinki Committee. The other body that performs such visits once every four years is the European Committee for the Prevention of Torture and Inhuman or Degrading Treatment or Punishment under the Council of Europe.
- In Lithuania, the regional office of the Global Initiative on Psychiatry, an international nongovernmental organization, and some other nongovernmental organizations perform inspections at their own initiative. The first patient attorney activity in mental health institutions started in Vilnius in 2006.

The review bodies have different remits.

- In Bulgaria, the aim of national monitoring is reporting and distributing reports and selecting strategic cases for litigation. The official accreditation procedure performed by the Ministry of Health includes a requirement to provide evidence of human rights protection, but in practice this is ineffective and formal.
- The former Yugoslav Republic of Macedonia has regulations addressing the protection of human rights of service users and institutions assigned to monitor their enforcement. However, there is an evident lack of implementation of the human rights issues in practice.
- In Switzerland, the supervisory and inspection agencies addressing the human rights aspects of the treatment of people with mental disorders are positioned at the cantonal level. The cantonal regulations differ significantly.
- In Georgia, the Public Monitoring Council under the Office of the Public Defender (Ombudsman) monitored all large psychiatric institutions in Georgia in 2006–2007 to examine issues related to living conditions in institutions, restraint of freedom and the use of involuntary measures. Twice a year the Public Defender prepares a report for the Parliament,

including the report of the Public Monitoring Council. The Medical Activity Regulation Agency of the Ministry of Health, Labour and Social Affairs examines the quality of psychiatric services and considers complaints.

- In the Russian Federation, the human rights protection of users admitted to mental health services is assessed in response to complaints but not yet on a regular basis. More than 100 nongovernmental organizations that have the duty to protect human rights and the interests of users of mental health services as stated in the statutes of these organizations carry out assessments. They usually carry out assessments in their regions. In December 2007, the Government of the Russian Federation decided to establish as of 2008 the Service for the Protection of Psychiatric Patients' Rights (implementing the corresponding article of the Law on Psychiatric Care (1993) that had not been implemented earlier). It will regularly assess and survey conditions in mental health hospitals.

External inspection of human rights protection of the users of mental health services in different types of facilities

The previous section indicates the existence of monitoring and inspection agencies and their roles. This section shows the proportion of countries that inspected facilities for people with mental disorders that had been subjected to external inspection of human rights protection of people using mental health services during the last year available. Countries were asked to provide data on annual external inspections in mental hospitals, community-based inpatient psychiatric units, community residential facilities and residential facilities that are not health care (social institutions).

Most countries report that mental hospitals had external inspection of human rights conditions at least annually (28 of the 42 countries that have mental hospitals). Information was not available for 10 of the 42 countries (Table 11.2).

The proportion of hospitals covered by inspections (in countries where inspections took place) varies. Twelve countries report that all their mental hospitals had external inspections during the last year available: Albania, Austria, Bosnia and Herzegovina (Republika Srpska), Bulgaria, Cyprus, Germany (Länder (regions): Berlin, Brandenburg, Mecklenburg–West Pomerania, Saxony and Schleswig-Holstein), Ireland, Portugal, Serbia, Spain (Castilla y León), the former Yugoslav Republic of Macedonia and the United Kingdom (England and Wales).

Other countries indicate that such inspections did take place, but not in all hospitals: Germany (Baden-Württemberg: 20%, Bavaria: 60%), Denmark (about 20%), Greece (10%), Russian Federation (about 5%) and Turkey (37.5%).

These lists show that some countries have regional variation, subject to their competence.

The frequency of inspections also varies from country to country.

- In France, the regional commissions on psychiatric hospitalization (CDHP) are in charge of visiting the mental hospitals at least twice a year.
- In Netherlands, the Health Care Inspectorate does not visit the mental hospitals on a regular yearly basis. Hospitals are inspected only when serious events have occurred or when they are included in a national assessment.

Fewer countries report that external inspection took place in community-based inpatient psychiatric units (17 of the 39 countries that had these facilities). Another 17 of 39 countries did not have information on whether such inspections were organized.

Seven countries report that inspections took place in all the community-based inpatient psychiatric units: Albania, Austria, Cyprus, Germany (Länder: Berlin, Brandenburg, Mecklenburg–West Pomerania, Saxony and Schleswig-Holstein), Ireland, the former Yugoslav Republic of Macedonia and United

Table11.2. External inspection of human rights protection of service users during the last year available in countries

Country	External inspection of human rights protection of service users in mental hospitals	External inspection of human rights protection of service users in community-based inpatient psychiatric units	External inspection of human rights protection of service users in community residential facilities	External inspection of human rights protection of service users in residential facilities that are not health care (social institutions)
Albania	Yes	Yes	No	Information not available
Austria	Yes	Yes	Yes	Yes
Azerbaijan	No	Not applicable	Not applicable	No
Belgium	Information not available	Information not available	Information not available	Information not available
Bosnia and Herzegovina				
Federation of Bosnia and Herzegovina	Information not available	No	Not applicable	Yes
Republika Srpska	Yes	Yes	Yes	Yes
Bulgaria	Yes	Information not available	Not applicable	Yes
Croatia	Yes	Yes	Not applicable	Yes
Cyprus	Yes	Yes	Yes	Yes
Czech Republic	Yes	Information not available	Information not available	Yes
Denmark	Yes	Yes	Yes	Yes
Estonia	Yes	Yes	Yes	Yes
Finland	Information not available	Information not available	Information not available	Information not available
France	Yes	Yes	Yes	Yes
Georgia	Yes	Not applicable	Not applicable	Yes
Germany	Yes	Yes	Yes	Yes
Greece	Yes	Yes	Yes	Yes
Hungary	Information not available	Information not available	Not applicable	Information not available
Ireland	Yes	Yes	Yes	Information not available
Israel	Information not available	Information not available	Not applicable	Information not available
Italy	Not applicable	Information not available	Information not available	Information not available
Latvia	Yes	No	Not applicable	Yes
Lithuania	Information not available	Information not available	Not applicable	No
Luxembourg	Information not available	Information not available	Information not available	Information not available
Malta	Yes	No	No	Not applicable
Moldova	Yes	Not applicable	Not applicable	Yes
Montenegro	Information not available	Not applicable	Not applicable	Information not available
Netherlands	No	No	No	No
Norway	Yes	Yes	Yes	Yes
Poland	Information not available	Information not available	No	Information not available
Portugal	Information not available	Information not available	Information not available	Information not available
Romania	Yes	Information not available	Information not available	Yes
Russian Federation	Yes	Information not available	Information not available	Information not available
Serbia	Yes	Yes	Yes	Yes
Slovakia	Yes	Yes	Not applicable	No
Slovenia	Yes	Information not available	Not applicable	Yes
Spain				
Castilla y León	Yes	Yes	Information not available	Information not available
Catalonia	No	No	No	No
Extremadura	No	No	No	No
Galicia	No	No	No	No
Murcia	Information not available	Information not available	Information not available	Information not available
Sweden	No	Information not available	Information not available	Information not available
Switzerland	Information not available	Information not available	Information not available	Information not available
The former Yugoslav Republic of Macedonia	Yes	Yes	Not applicable	Not applicable
Turkey	Yes	Information not available	Not applicable	Information not available
United Kingdom				
England and Wales	Yes	Yes	Yes	Yes
Scotland	Information not available	Information not available	Information not available	Information not available
Uzbekistan	Yes	Yes	Not applicable	Information not available

Yes ■ No ■ Not applicable ■ Information not available

Kingdom (England and Wales), overlapping considerably with mental hospital inspections.

Countries in which external inspections covered a limited number of community psychiatric inpatient units are: Bosnia and Herzegovina (Republika Srpska) – 80% of facilities; Greece – 10%; Spain (Castilla y León) – 6–7%.

External inspection of community residential facilities took place in 12 of the 24 countries with such facilities. As many as 10 of 24 countries with such facilities did not provide information (Fig. 11.9).

External inspection covered all the community residential facilities in Austria, Bosnia and Herzegovina (Republika Srpska), Germany, Ireland, The former Yugoslav Republic of Macedonia and the United Kingdom (England and Wales).

- In Austria, residents' advocates in residential facilities have to be informed about any restriction of liberty and also have the right to perform unannounced inspections (legal regulation within the law on restriction of liberty in residential facilities).
- In Denmark, the municipalities inspect the community-based residential facilities and the social institutions, but the frequency of inspection is up to the municipality.
- In Germany, the Medical Advisory Board of the Health Insurance Funds (MDK) has been obligated by the Social Code to monitor long-term care facilities since 1996. This can take place without prior notice but is not expected to be undertaken annually. In addition, the Nursing Home Act prescribes monitoring activities that are to be undertaken at least once a year by the responsible authorities. The authorities responsible for overseeing such homes can vary depending on the Land but are usually local authorities.
- In Italy, some inspections have been conducted at the local level, but information is not available on the proportion of facilities inspected.

External inspections of social institutions were organized in 18 of the 41 countries with such facilities. While 5 countries report that these institutions have not been inspected, another 16 countries could not provide information (Fig. 11.10). The lack of information can be explained by the fact that social care institutions in most countries are not under the authority of the health ministries, and inspections (if organized) are therefore not reported to the health authorities.

In Austria, Bosnia and Herzegovina (Federation of Bosnia and Herzegovina and Republika Srpska), Germany and the United Kingdom (England and Wales), all such facilities were inspected in the last available year.

In Azerbaijan, the European Committee for the Prevention of Torture and Inhuman or Degrading Treatment or Punishment under the Council of Europe inspected two mental health hospitals in 2006 and found that human rights are commonly violated in psychiatric institutions.

Representation of service users and carers on review bodies

Since the monitoring and inspection bodies focus on the experiences of service users and carers involved with mental health services, their inclusion on visiting teams would add great value and credibility. In the Mental Health Declaration for Europe, Member States commit themselves to ensuring that users and carers are involved in reviewing and inspecting mental health services. This section reports on national practices.

Of the 29 countries reporting that external inspections took place last year, 9 indicated that users were represented on the review bodies assessing the human rights in these facilities and 6 indicated that family members or carers were involved in the inspections (Table 11.3).

Users' involvement in human rights inspections in different countries includes the following examples.

Table 11.3. Representation of service users and carers in national and regional review bodies assessing the human rights protection of the users of mental health services in groups of countries

Representation in national and regional review bodies	EU		EU15		New EU countries since 2004		Israel, Norway and Switzerland		South-eastern Europe		CIS		Total	
	No.	%	No.	%	No.	%	No.	%	No.	%	No.	%	No.	%
Users														
Yes	5	19	5	33	0	0	0	0	2	29	2	40	9	21
No	16	59	6	40	10	83	0	0	4	57	3	60	23	55
Information not available	6	22	4	27	2	17	3	100	1	14	0	0	10	24
Carers														
Yes	3	11	3	20	0	0	1	33	1	14	1	20	6	14
No	18	67	8	53	10	83	0	0	5	71	4	80	27	64
Information not available	6	22	4	27	2	17	2	67	1	14	0	0	9	21

- In Albania, the mental hospital in Elbasan has been visited by a team of experts, and a user representative has been part of the team.
- In Austria, patients' advocates have a permanent office in each psychiatric hospital with constant monitoring of conditions (legal regulation within the Law on Civil Commitment (Unterbringungsgesetz)).
- Bulgaria has no users' organizations; during inspections they are always interviewed in detail, but "they do not want to be involved in such activities because of the additional trauma".
- In Denmark, service users are not represented on the review bodies. However, members of the national-level review body are elected members of Folketinget (parliament), who thus – in a sense – inspect on behalf of the population. Service users are interviewed during the inspections. Members of the other type of national-level review body (from the Ombudsman) consist of civil servants. During these inspections, service users are also interviewed, in private if they so wish.
- In Georgia, users of services participated in monitoring of only three psychiatric hospitals. They also participated in designing the assessment of these three services, which the European Commission supported financially.
- In Germany, the home review board established by the Law on Homes, Residential Homes for the Elderly and Nursing Homes for Older Residents interviews both the residents and the home advisory boards. Every resident and the home advisory boards can appeal to the home monitoring authorities. The Medical Advisory Service of the Health Insurance Funds also involves service users in their reviews.
- In the United Kingdom (England and Wales), service users are always involved as members of the review teams.

Examples of carers' involvement in human rights inspections in different countries include the following.

- In France, family and carers are actively involved in inspections and other activities related to health services for people with mental health problems, particularly the National Union of Friends and Families of People with Mental Illness (UNAFAM).
- In the United Kingdom (England and Wales), carers are also always involved as members of the review teams.
- Bulgaria and Romania report that carers are not involved in inspections organized in mental health facilities because "they do not want to be involved". There are no carers' associations in either of these countries.

Availability of protocols for involuntary admission, restraint and violence management

Monitoring and inspection is facilitated by the availability of standards of good practice, such as protocols that have been developed

Table 11.4. Availability of protocols for involuntary admission, restraint and violence management in groups of countries

Protocols	EU		EU15		New EU countries since 2004		Israel, Norway and Switzerland		South-eastern Europe		CIS		Total	
	No.	%	No.	%	No.	%	No.	%	No.	%	No.	%	No.	%
Involuntary admission														
Yes	23	85	14	93	9	75	2	67	7	100	4	80	36	86
No	4	15	1	7	3	25	0	0	0	0	1	20	5	12
Information not available	0	0	0	0	0	0	1	33	0	0	0	0	1	2
Restraint														
Yes	23	85	15	100	8	67	2	67	7	100	3	60	35	83
No	4	15	0	0	4	33	0	0	0	0	2	40	6	14
Information not available	0	0	0	0	0	0	1	33	0	0	0	0	1	2
Violence management														
Yes	16	59	12	80	4	33	2	67	6	86	1	20	25	60
No	7	26	1	7	6	50	0	0	1	14	3	60	11	26
Information not available	4	15	2	13	2	17	1	33	0	0	1	20	6	14

nationally, regionally or locally. Especially relevant for human rights monitoring are protocols for involuntary admission, restraint and violence management.

The large majority of countries indicate they have protocols for both involuntary admission (36 of 42 countries) and for restraint (35 of 42 countries) (Table 11.4). Protocols for violence management are available in 25 of 42 countries.

The protocols for involuntary admission and restraint are typically specified in legal documents, for example:

- in Finland, in the Mental Health Act No. 1116/1990;
- in France, in specific legislation for the protection of individual liberties, sections L.3212-1 et seq., L.3213-1 et seq. of the Public Health Code;
- in Georgia, in the Law on Psychiatric Care, Article 18 and Ministry of Health, Labour and Social Affairs Decree No. 87/n;
- in Ireland, in the Mental Health Act 2001, which regulates involuntary admissions, and the Mental Health Commission rules, which govern the use of seclusion and mechanical means of bodily restraint; and
- in the Russian Federation, in the Law on Psychiatric Care.

The presence of laws and protocols cannot always be assumed to imply familiarity or adherence. Some countries admit that these protocols are not always followed.

- Bosnia and Herzegovina (Federation of Bosnia and Herzegovina): it is not clear to what degree protocols are implemented.
- The former Yugoslav Republic of Macedonia: legislation regulates the involuntary admission, but the remaining problem is the use of this regulation in everyday practice.

The meaning of protocols for managing violence differs across countries. Thus, in some countries they refer to procedural requirements included in legal documents (such as Denmark), whereas in others they are policy documents specifying practice (such as in the United Kingdom (England and Wales)).

In Denmark, every time a person is subjected to involuntary admission, treatment or restraint, a separate protocol has to be filled out, as required by the Mental Health Act. This protocol is recorded in the patient record, and all the records are available at any time for review or inspection in the department for the staff, the regional medical officer and other inspection authorities. All this information is also reported to the National Board of Health, which prepares annual reports that are published on its web site. Significant efforts are made to validate the data collected at the national level. This system ensures systematic monitoring of involuntary admission, treatment and restraint.

Registration of involuntary admission, restraint and seclusion

Most countries report that involuntary admission, restraint and seclusion are registered (37 of 42, 34 of 42 and 26 of 42 countries, respectively) (Table 11.5). The manner in which involuntary admission and restraint are registered varies considerably from country to country.

The following are examples of registration of involuntary admission.

- In Bulgaria, the registered cases of involuntary admission are not available at the national level because of the lack of a national information system that could analyse such data. The cases of restraint and seclusion are kept in the hospital records but are not processed at the national level.
- In the Czech Republic, the data on involuntary admission are not collected centrally but only registered in patients' documentation.
- In Georgia, involuntary admission, restraint and seclusion are recorded in separate wards only in the medical documentation completed by nurses. They are not gathered at the level of hospital administration.
- In the Netherlands, the Health Care Inspectorate, designated by law as the registering agent, registers involuntary admission at the national level.

The following are examples of registration of restraint.

- In Austria, restraint is only registered at the hospital level.
- In Bosnia and Herzegovina (Federation of Bosnia and Herzegovina), each incident of restraint is registered in a nursing report.
- In Croatia, restraint is registered in hospital and court documents.
- In Lithuania, restraint is recorded in the medical case record of the patient.
- In the Netherlands, restraint is registered at the institute or hospital.
- In the Russian Federation, restraint and the reasons are registered in the patient's medical records.

Seclusion is registered in a similar manner as restraint. Three countries indicate that seclusion of users of mental health services does not take place.

Table 11.5. Registration of involuntary admission, restraint and seclusion in groups of countries

	EU		EU15		New EU countries since 2004		Israel, Norway and Switzerland		South-eastern Europe		CIS		Total	
Registration	No.	%	No.	%	No.	%	No.	%	No.	%	No.	%	No.	%
Involuntary admission														
Yes	24	89	15	100	9	75	2	67	6	86	5	100	37	88
No	2	7	0	0	2	17	0	0	0	0	0	0	2	5
Information not available	1	4	0	0	1	8	1	33	1	14	0	0	3	7
Restraint														
Yes	22	81	15	100	7	58	2	67	6	86	4	80	34	81
No	4	15	0	0	4	33	0	0	0	0	1	20	5	12
Information not available	1	4	0	0	1	8	1	33	1	14	0	0	3	7
Seclusion														
Yes	16	59	11	73	5	42	2	67	6	86	2	40	26	62
No	4	15	0	0	4	33	0	0	0	0	3	60	7	17
Not applicable	3	11	2	13	1	8	0	0	0	0	0	0	3	7
Information not available	4	15	2	13	2	17	1	33	1	14	0	0	6	14

Table 11.6. Availability of rates of involuntary admission, restraint and seclusion in countries

Country	Rates of involuntary admission available	Rates of restraint available	Rates of seclusion available
Albania	No	No	No
Austria	Yes	No	No
Azerbaijan	No	No	No
Belgium	Yes	No	No
Bosnia and Herzegovina			
Federation of Bosnia and Herzegovina	Yes	Yes	Not applicable
Republika Srpska	Yes	Yes	Yes
Bulgaria	No	No	No
Croatia	No	No	No
Cyprus	Yes	Yes	No
Czech Republic	No	No	No
Denmark	Yes	Yes	Not applicable
Estonia	No	No	No
Finland	Yes	Yes	Yes
France	Yes	No	No
Georgia	No	No	No
Germany	Yes	Yes	No
Greece	No	No	No
Hungary	Yes	No	No
Ireland	Yes	No	No
Israel	No	No	No
Italy	Yes	No	Not applicable
Latvia	No	No	No
Lithuania	Yes	No	No
Luxembourg	No	No	No
Malta	Yes	No	No
Moldova	Yes	Yes	No
Montenegro	No	No	No
Netherlands	Yes	Yes	Yes
Norway	No	No	No
Poland	Yes	No	Yes
Portugal	Yes	No	No
Romania	No	No	No
Russian Federation	Yes	No	No
Serbia	Yes	Yes	Yes
Slovakia	No	No	No
Slovenia	No	No	No
Spain			
Castilla y León	No	No	No
Catalonia	No	No	No
Extremadura	No	No	No
Galicia	No	No	No
Murcia	No	No	No
Sweden	Yes	No	No
Switzerland	No	No	No
The former Yugoslav Republic of Macedonia	Yes	Yes	Yes
Turkey	No	No	No
United Kingdom			
England and Wales	Yes	Yes	Yes
Scotland	No	No	No
Uzbekistan	No	No	No

Yes No Not applicable

- In Bosnia and Herzegovina (Federation of Bosnia and Herzegovina), there is no seclusion in institutions.
- In Denmark, seclusion is not permitted according to law, except in the one existing high-security department for people with mental disorders that have been convicted of a crime and committed by the courts as being highly dangerous, where it is allowed to lock the door of the patient's own room at night and for brief periods in the daytime. This department has 30 beds.
- In Italy seclusion is not allowed in public services.

Although involuntary admission, restraint and seclusion are registered in some way in most countries, this does not mean that countries can make these data available. Only 22 of 42 countries produced rates for involuntary admission, 10 of 42 for restraint and 7 of 42 for seclusion (Table 11.6).

Although these countries produced rates on involuntary admission, restraint and seclusion, the way data had been collected and presented was quite inconsistent across countries, and publication in such a format would be misleading.

One intriguing example of feedback from a non-EU country stated that "patients are influenced to sign the document regarding their agreement with voluntary hospitalization". This country did not report any involuntary admissions.

Right to access to legal representation free of charge for people committed involuntarily

If human rights are to be respected and reinforced, people committed involuntarily require the right of appeal and access to legal representation. Considering that many such people and their relatives are unable to afford to pay such representation from personal means, such representation should be made available for free at request, and these people need to be informed of their rights.

The meaning of "right" can be ambiguous in this context. Most countries report that people involuntary committed to mental health facilities have the right to access to free legal representation. An exception is Malta. Israel could not provide information on this issue. However, the enforcement of this right is poor in some countries.

- In Bulgaria, the formal recognition of this right is extremely ineffective. In practice, the lawyers do not take any active role in the hearings. They are only present and often have never talked to their clients.
- In Georgia, people admitted involuntary have this right in principle, but there are no legal services that would not charge these people, and the large majority cannot afford to hire a lawyer
- In the former Yugoslav Republic of Macedonia, even if there are formal instruments that should ensure this right, there are very few examples of it being respected in practice.
- In Turkey people involuntarily committed have the right to access to free legal representation. But there is no information as to whether anybody has exercised this right.

Main activities initiated and developed since 2005 related to protecting the human rights of people with mental health problems

- Albania: regular inspection of mental health services; raised awareness of the mass media to the human rights of people with mental disorders; new regulation of the mental health services.
- Bosnia and Herzegovina (Republika Srpska): establishment of commissions for inspection of psychiatric hospitals and monitoring the implementation of the Mental Health Law. Inclusion of users in commissions. Establishment of users' associations.
- Denmark: the National Board of Health, the administrative regions and the patient organizations have created a nationwide project using the Breakthrough Series

method to develop a culture at the hospital units to improve the quality of compulsory treatment. A new Mental Health Care Act improves statutory rights. The Act was passed in 2006 and entered into force on 1 January 2007.

- Estonia: a review mechanism by the Chancellor of Justice was implemented in 2003; the Code of Civil Procedure has changed the procedure for involuntary admissions, mainly endorsing safeguards since 2006.
- The former Yugoslav Republic of Macedonia: the Parliament adopted the Mental Health Law in June 2006, focusing mainly on human rights issues.
- Georgia: in 2005, the Public Monitoring Council was established under the Office of the Public Defender (Ombudsman). In 2006, Parliament adopted the new Law on Psychiatric Care.
- Ireland: the Mental Health Act 2001 was implemented on a phased basis. It became fully operational in November 2006.
- Montenegro: adoption and enforcement of the Law on the Protection of and the Exercise of the Rights of People with Mental Disorders.
- Norway: an action plan for reducing the use of involuntary treatment in 2006; initiatives for an Anti-Discrimination Act that entered into force on 2006; a national strategy to reduce social inequality in health from 2006.
- Poland: amendments to the Mental Health Act concerning the ombudsmen of the rights of psychiatric hospital patients (2005).
- Romania: implementation rules for the Mental Health Law (2 May 2006) and a Ministerial Order for monitoring human rights in psychiatric hospitals (27 March 2006).
- Sweden: introducing involuntary treatment in outpatient care.
- United Kingdom (England and Wales): passage of new national mental health legislation in 2007 includes, for example, rights to independent advocacy. A new Mental Capacity Act in 2006.

Discussion

Human rights protection is a central issue in the care of people with mental health problems, who are vulnerable and exposed to neglect and abuse. Findings on monitoring, the presence of protocols and the availability of national data for involuntary admission, restraint and seclusion show considerable variation and are not always reassuring.

The proportion of countries reporting the presence of inspection bodies is high, and many performed a wide range of functions, especially in the EU15 countries. Many of these countries seem to have invested in intensive systems of monitoring and inspection. However, even in these countries the representation of users and carers on visits to mental facilities, a commitment in the Mental Health Declaration for Europe, was far from standard.

Some countries reporting positively on the existence of inspection bodies and representation of users and carers acknowledge that the practice is very limited. For example, in some instances a single visit was made to a hospital, organized by a nongovernmental organization. However, the recognition that involving users and carers is good practice is positive, and it is to be hoped that countries can learn from these examples and build on them. The constructive role of many nongovernmental organizations in this field should be acknowledged.

Of concern is that only a few countries provided data on rates of involuntarily admission, restraint or seclusion, even though more than 70% of the countries report that national and regional review bodies are assigned to review these functions and register them in some form.

This report indicates that protocols, particularly for involuntary admission and restraint but less so for violence management, are widely available across the European Region. The next question is the comparability and quality of these protocols and the degree of their distribution and adherence.

These findings show that further efforts are needed to collect basic data to allow more in-depth analysis of comparative data and dissemination of good practices related to safeguarding the human rights of people with mental disorders. This could include reviewing procedures to prevent poor practices and abuse related to involuntary admission and involuntary treatment and reviewing the availability and effectiveness of alternatives to restraint or seclusion.

Finally, access and affordability to legal representation is very poor in some countries, despite the legal right to such free legal representation. Without such representation, the people with mental health problems are unlikely to be in a position to enforce their rights, and this needs to be redressed urgently.

Many countries are making progress in this area, and it is to be hoped that these data will stimulate countries toward further progress.

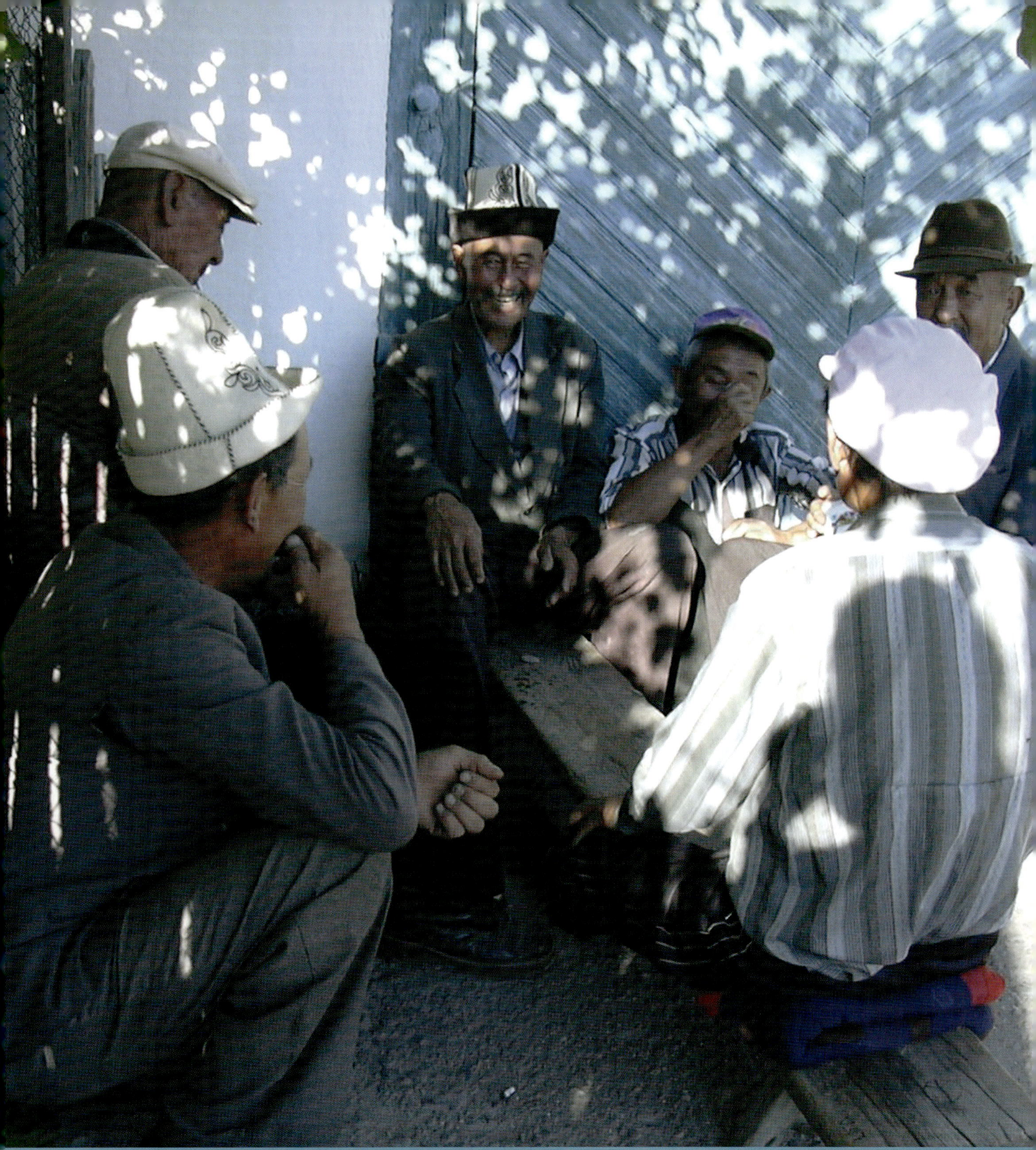

PHOTO © MELITTA JAKAB

“Findings confirm that international collaboration could be productive in information and research”

12. Information and research on mental health

The governance of health systems relies on a valid data set to monitor trends, especially at a time of reform when input, process, output and outcome measures may indicate the success or failure and a need for intervention at the policy level[1]. Eurostat collects some variables at the international level on behalf of the European Commission. Research programmes such as the European Study of the Epidemiology of Mental Disorders (ESEMeD) project collect data for some detailed but more limited data sets[2].

Earlier chapters in this report identified some major gaps in information and needs for research. This chapter outlines the present status of information systems at the local or national level in European countries. A distinction has been made between health and other systems. Since community-based mental health services rely heavily for effective functioning on partnerships across sectors, it would have been ideal to know about compatibility, but this question was not considered realistic.

This chapter also reports on research investment. The objective of community-based mental health care is to develop services responding to the needs of the population and individuals. This requires epidemiological data and needs assessments to inform policy-makers and planners. Finally, the survey enquired about agencies in countries responsible for producing and disseminating guidelines, encouraging consistent standards of practice.

Information on mental health

Data collection systems in mental health facilities

Nearly all countries collect a minimum set of data based on defined indicators from mental hospitals, and most of the countries also collect data from the community mental health sector (Table 12.1). Information on whether data are collected from the social care sector is not available in 15 of 42 countries. There seems to be a surprising inverse correlation between the complexity of the social care system and the collection of data in the social care sector. Thus, social care data are more available in the lower-income countries in the CIS and south-eastern Europe than in EU countries. The reason is that data collected in the CIS countries, south-eastern Europe and many of the EU countries joining since 2004 are simple, mostly consisting of numbers of residents in institutional social care settings, as explained in the country examples.

The following are examples of country activities.

- Finland: in practice data are collected very well in institutional settings but are less reliable and extensive in primary health care, basic social services and community-based mental health care.
- Georgia: social care residences do not complete special statistical forms but regularly write brief reports to the Ministry of Health. At the end of each year, all mental health facilities send a special statistical form to the Centre for Disease Control and Medical Statistics of the Ministry of Health.
- Germany: in hospital practice, the BaDo (basic documentation) system has established itself as a kind of standard, although it is seldom implemented in the recommended form in hospitals. The situation has become even more confusing, since the items in the most widespread version of BaDo (DBPPN Version – A, E, ZA and ZE items) have been changed repeatedly in the past years. Not only for this reason but also because of the particular interests of the individual software providers that work with the hospitals, most of the BaDo applications have compatibility problems with other BaDo sets. More uniformity has been achieved only in certain geographical areas (Baden-Württemberg, for example) because of obligations concerning documentation.

1 *Health statistics. Key data on health 2002. Data 1970–2001.* Luxembourg, Office for Official Publications of the European Communities, 2002. Health in Europe. Results from 1997–2000 surveys. Luxembourg, Office for Official Publications of the European Communities, 2003.

2 Alonso J et al. Use of mental health services in Europe: results from the European Study of the Epidemiology of Mental Disorders (ESEMeD) project. *Acta Psychiatrica Scandinavica*, 2004, 109(Suppl 420):47–54.

Table 12.1. Collection of a formally defined mental health data from different sectors (minimum data set) in groups of countries

Sectors collecting data	EU		EU15		New EU countries since 2004		Israel, Norway and Switzerland		South-eastern Europe		CIS		Total	
	No.	%	No.	%	No.	%	No.	%	No.	%	No.	%	No.	%
Hospital														
Yes	26	96	15	100	11	92	3	100	6	86	5	100	40	95
No	1	4	0	0	1	8	0	0	0	0	0	0	1	2
Information not available	0	0	0	0	0	0	0	0	1	14	0	0	1	2
Community mental health														
Yes	22	81	12	80	10	83	2	67	5	71	4	80	33	79
No	1	4	0	0	1	8	0	0	0	0	0	0	1	2
Information not available	4	15	3	20	1	8	1	33	2	29	1	20	8	19
Social services														
Yes	13	48	7	47	6	50	2	67	4	57	4	80	23	55
No	3	11	0	0	3	25	0	0	0	0	1	20	4	10
Information not available	11	41	8	53	3	25	1	33	3	43	0	0	15	36

- Greece: although there has been defined a list of indicators since 1996 (DATAPSY), such data are not collected.
- Hungary: there is a unified database within certain clinics and hospitals but no nationwide network (with all mental health facilities included in the country).
- Lithuania: the Health Information Centre under the Ministry of Health collects and analyzes statistical information about the health status of the population and the activity and resources of health care institutions, including human resources. It also coordinates a public health monitoring programme that includes mental health.
- Poland: the Institute of Psychiatry and Neurology has collected and published annually (statistical yearbook) data on mental health services, including their human and material resources since 1968.
- Russian Federation: an official reporting form for primary registration is completed in the mental health institution (dispensaries and psychiatric hospitals) for every person receiving mental health care.
- Serbia: the data are regularly collected in official reports made quarterly. Each institution submits data to the Republic Institute for Public Health.
- United Kingdom (Scotland): there are clinical data standards for: 1) encounter and intervention recording in community mental health services; and 2) for clinical psychiatric discharge summaries. These are no minimum data sets because collection of each of the data items they contain is not mandated. However, they do mandate that when a data item is collected, it must be collected in the nationally agreed format. See the Health and social care data dictionary[3].

Reports covering mental health data

Reports covering mental health data are being published by or on behalf of the government health department in 34 of 42 countries (Table 12.2). Some countries produce reports that include analysis of the findings, whereas others release statistical data.

Some countries publish dedicated mental health reports (such as Austria, Germany, Ireland, the Netherlands and the United Kingdom (England and Wales)), and other countries present mental health data as part of overall health reports (such as Bosnia and Herzegovina (Federation of Bosnia and Herzegovina), Bosnia and Herzegovina (Republika Srpska), Bulgaria, Georgia, Russian Federation and the former Yugoslav Republic of Macedonia).

3 *Health and social care data dictionary*. Edinburgh, Information Services Division, NHS National Services Scotland, 2008 (http://www.datadictionaryadmin.scot.nhs.uk/isddd/9215.html, accessed 8 May 2008).

Table 12.2. Availability of regular reports covering mental health data published by or on behalf of the government health department in groups of countries

Sectors collecting data	EU		EU15		New EU countries since 2004		Israel, Norway and Switzerland		South-eastern Europe		CIS		Total	
	No.	%	No.	%	No.	%	No.	%	No.	%	No.	%	No.	%
Yes	23	85	12	80	11	92	3	100	4	57	4	80	34	81
No	4	15	3	20	1	8	0	0	2	29	1	20	7	17
Information not available	0	0	0	0	0	0	0	0	1	14	0	0	1	2

Research on mental health

Funding of mental health research

Public money is funding research in mental health in 25 of 42 countries (Fig. 12.1). Information on the proportion of the overall health research budget allocated to mental health research is not available in 27 of 42 countries. In countries for which information is available funding varies considerably, both in absolute terms and as a proportion of the overall research budget (Tables 12.3 and 12.4). The tables below show that only the EU15 countries, Israel, Norway and Switzerland could afford to invest in research, and even in these countries the large majority of countries did not provide any information.

- Switzerland: the Swiss National Science Foundation database system does not allow for segregation of the above mentioned categories. In 2006, 59 research projects on mental health–related topics – including basic brain research – were up and running, for a total of Sw.fr. 17.3 million (average Sw.fr. 293 000 per project).
- United Kingdom (England and Wales): There is a government-funded national mental health research network. Research to better understand mental illness and the impact of mental health services continues to be a priority for the Department of Health. In March 2007, the National Director of Mental Health announced £1 million in new funding for research to support implementation of the Mental Health Act, and in April 2007 the Department of Health announced a further £45 million for research into mental health, such as services in primary care and improving physical health for people with severe mental illness. The Department of Health has already awarded more than £7.4 million to mental health trusts in the current fiscal year through the new National Institute for Health Research funding streams. The National Institute for Health Research is, and intends to continue to be, a major funder of mental health research.
- Netherlands: 368 research projects in mental health and addiction funded by ZonMw (organization for health research and development in the Netherlands) with average budgets of €100 000 per year = €37 million on a total budget of €100 million.
- Germany: research focus on psychotherapy (eating disorders, social phobias, attention deficit disorder, anxiety disorders and psychosis), 2006–2010, €13 million; Competency Network on Depression and Suicidality, 1999–2008, €15.1 million; Competency Network on Schizophrenia, 1999–2009, €14.5 million; Competency Network on Dementia, 2002–2007, €12.7 million.

Fig. 12.1. Allocation of public funds to mental health research in countries

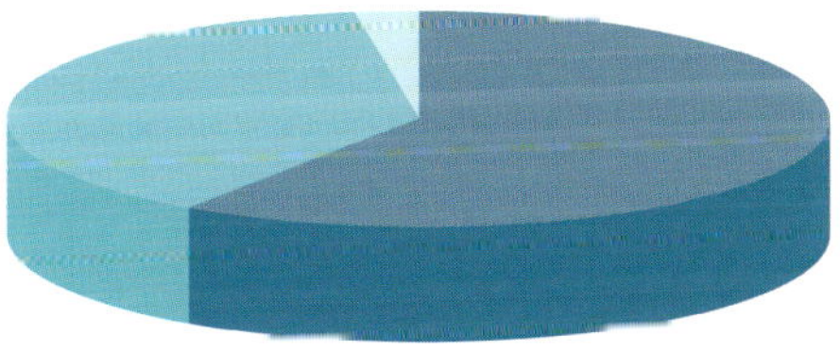

Yes:
Belgium, Bosnia and Herzegovina (Federation of Bosnia and Herzegovina and Republika Srpska), Bulgaria, Croatia, Czech Republic, Denmark, Estonia, Finland, France, Germany, Ireland, Israel, Italy, Lithuania, Luxembourg, Netherlands, Norway, Portugal, Moldova, Russian Federation, Slovenia, Spain (Castilla y León and Catalonia), Sweden, Switzerland, United Kingdom (England and Wales and Scotland)

No:
Albania, Austria, Azerbaijan, Cyprus, Georgia, Greece, Hungary, Latvia, Malta, Poland, Romania, Serbia, Slovakia, Spain (Extremadura, Galicia, Murcia), the former Yugoslav Republic of Macedonia, Turkey, Uzbekistan

Information not available:
Montenegro

Table 12.3. Allocation of public funds to mental health research in groups of countries

Allocation of public funds	EU		EU15		New EU countries since 2004		Israel, Norway and Switzerland		South-eastern Europe		CIS		Total	
	No.	%	No.	%	No.	%	No.	%	No.	%	No.	%	No.	%
Yes	18	67	13	87	5	42	3	100	2	29	2	40	25	60
No	9	33	2	13	7	58	0	0	4	57	3	60	16	38
Information not available	0	0	0	0	0	0	0	0	1	14	0	0	1	2

Table 12.4. Proportion of the overall health research budget allocated to mental health research in countries

Country	Proportion (%)	Comments
Bulgaria	6	Planned but not spent in 2006. The budget for 2007 was the same but the money was not available.
Czech Republic	3.8	Estimate
Germany	9	
Ireland	18.5	Includes €5 million allocated to autism research in 2006. The total amount for new research in mental health was about €6 million.
Israel	7.7	
Italy	5	Data refer only to research funding of the Research Department of the Ministry of Health.
Poland	10	Rough estimate for 2003
Spain (Castilla y Léon)	17	
Switzerland	12.9	Global Swiss National Science Foundation budget: CHF 430.8 million. Biomedical research: CHF 134.2. million. Mental-health-related research: CHF 17.3 million´. Federal Social Insurance Office disability research programme: CHF 3 million for three years, of which CHF 1 million (33.3%) is research into mental causes of disability
United Kingdom		
England and Wales	About 7–10	£40.2 million (additional £34 million for neuroscience research). Exact total spending on health research is not available.
Scotland	7.5	Chief Scientist Office (£4 million); Health Department Analytical Services Division of the Scottish Executive: two discrete programmes of research (about £650 000 annually).

Table 12.5. Allocation of mental health research budget to different types of research in countries

Country	Proportion of mental health research budget (%)		
	Service research	Health promotion and disorder prevention	Other areas (%)
Bulgaria	6	Information not available	Information not available
Georgia	0	0	0
Israel	0	28	72
Italy	35	15	50
Switzerland	80	0	20
United Kingdom			
England and Wales	31	4	65
Scotland	13 (Chief Scientist Office) 0 (Health Department Analytical Services Division of the Scottish Executive)	0 (Chief Scientist Office) 66 (Health Department Analytical Services Division of the Scottish Executive)	87 (Chief Scientist Office) 33 (Health Department Analytical Services Division of the Scottish Executive)

Box 12.1. Producing and disseminating evidence-based treatment guidelines for mental health in the Netherlands

The National Steering Committee for Multidisciplinary Guidelines Development in Mental Health Care has been in operation since January 1999. This Committee comprises the professional associations for primary care doctors, psychiatrists, psychotherapists, psychologists and nurses. The Committee is supported by the Dutch Institute for Health Care Improvement and the Trimbos Institute (Netherlands Institute of Mental Health and Addiction, www.trimbos.nl). The Steering Committee is further supported by an Advisory Board comprising employers in mental health care, health insurance funds, the national government, universities and the Netherlands Health Care Inspectorate. The Steering Committee has (advisory) subcommittees for client involvement and for implementation. The Steering Committee is responsible for developing and implementing multidisciplinary guidelines in collaboration with the Trimbos Institute and the Dutch Institute for Health Care Improvement. The secretariat of the Committee is at the Trimbos Institute.

Countries struggled to answer how the mental health research budget is distributed across different research areas such as mental health services, mental health promotion, mental disorder prevention or other research areas. About 80% of the countries reported that this kind of information is not available (Table 12.5).

Organizations responsible for producing and disseminating evidence-based treatment guidelines for mental health

Most countries (29 of 43) have assigned an organization or organizations responsible for producing and disseminating evidence based treatment guidelines for mental health (Box 12.1, Fig. 12.2).

Fig. 12.2. Presence of an organization responsible for producing and disseminating evidence-based treatment guidelines for mental health in countries

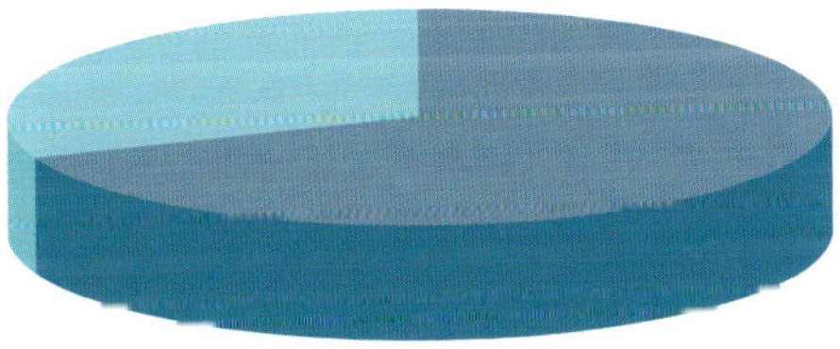

Yes:
Belgium, Bosnia and Herzegovina (Federation of Bosnia and Herzegovina and Republika Srpska), Bulgaria, Croatia, Czech Republic, Estonia, Finland, France, Georgia, Germany, Hungary, Ireland, Israel, Italy, Latvia, Lithuania, Luxembourg, Netherlands, Norway, Poland, Romania, Russian Federation, Serbia, Slovenia, Spain (Castilla y León, Catalonia, Extremadura, Galicia and Murcia), Sweden, the former Yugoslav Republic of Macedonia, United Kingdom (England and Wales and Scotland), Uzbekistan

No:
Albania, Austria, Azerbaijan , Cyprus, Denmark, Greece, Malta, Montenegro, Portugal, Moldova, Slovakia, Switzerland, Turkey

Denmark has a national policy of producing guidelines for all common health conditions, including mental health. In practice, the responsibility for producing guidelines is not assigned to one single institution. Various institutions such as the National Board of Health or professional societies have produced guidelines for several mental health conditions.

Discussion

This chapter reinforces the major divide across the European Region between countries with well-developed information systems that also invest in research and dissemination, typically the EU15 countries, and the countries that do not. If these data were cross-tabulated with the presence of community services and diversity of workforce, a clear correlation would be found.

All countries systematically collect hospital information data. Data on community mental health and social care activities are less comprehensively collected. These data sets are probably not linked in many countries, possibly even using incompatible software. This is a great challenge for the future.

This survey mostly provides qualitative data, but the research investment in some EU countries is higher than the total mental health budget of some lower-income countries in the European Region. Slightly surprising is the lack of information about investment in specific categories, possibly due to decentralized research funding bodies.

Many countries have agencies responsible for producing and disseminating evidence-based treatment guidelines for mental health. Considering the few countries investing heavily in research, most countries probably have no access to original research. This suggests that most agencies are analysing identical research, presumably to publish comparable treatment guidelines. Although some adaptation to the unique characteristics of individual countries is essential, if only for translation purposes, and since implementation relies on local ownership, a national role is justifiable, but there may be a place for close collaboration that could deliver considerable gains in quality and efficiency.

These findings confirm that international collaboration could be productive in information and research. However, the challenges of the availability and reliability of data are major obstacles, as has been illustrated by past attempts. The most promising area is probably identifying and disseminating good evidence, allowing local agencies to adapt this for local implementation.

"This report is the first ambitious attempt to bring together data on mental health policy and practice from across the European Region of WHO"

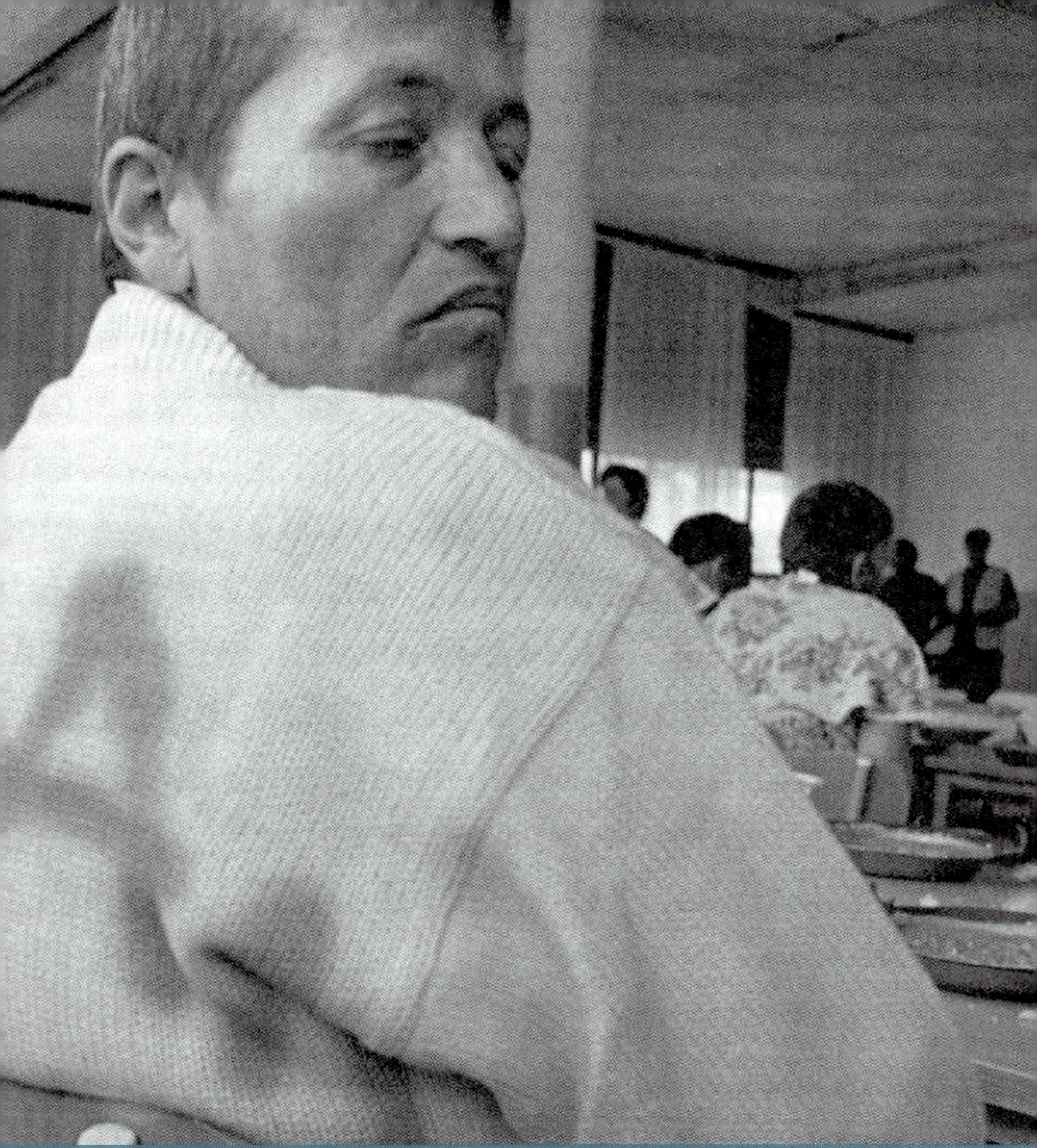

PHOTO © LILIANA URBINA

"If one word could summarize this report, it would be diversity"

13. Conclusion

This first European baseline survey, conducted by the WHO Regional Office for Europe and co-funded by the European Commission, offers an overview of the status of mental health activities in the WHO European Region. A large majority of the European Member States, 42 countries representing every part of the Region, completed the questionnaire. The report, therefore, offers an impression of the state of development in countries across the European Region and permits some cautious analysis of the state of mental health policies and programmes.

The WHO Regional Office for Europe coordinated the data collection, working closely with its counterparts in countries. Data were produced on behalf of the health ministries of countries and usually involved several departments within the ministries. Submissions were checked and queried repeatedly, but the resulting data are the responsibility of countries and have not been independently validated or cross-checked. This would have been very challenging in any case, since no independent sources exist apart from very few research projects that have focused on narrow fields also covered in this report such as number of beds and admissions or levels of funding, using different methods.

Overall, the chapters present a picture of progress in many of the areas covered by the Mental Health Declaration for Europe and Mental Health Action Plan for Europe. Some European countries lead the world in the vision and quality of activities. The large majority of countries now have mental health policies and legislation, and many, but not all, countries are making some progress towards implementing community based mental health services. The role of primary care in the care of people with mental health problems is growing, and partnerships with other agencies are being established. Most countries are creating an increasingly diverse and competent workforce. Countries are gradually accepting the involvement of service users and carers as good practice, and most countries are establishing programmes for the social inclusion of service users, if often initially on a small and local scale.

None of these developments is homogeneous across the Region. If one word could summarize this report, it would be diversity. Many sentences and tables in the chapters are characterized by diverse differences.

Diverse differences can be exemplified by the numbers of psychiatrists, which most countries were able to provide reliably, since registries for this specialist profession that requires licensing and certification exist everywhere. The rates are diverse, varying more than 10-fold across the European Region. Nevertheless, there is more behind these data than diversity of rates. Psychiatrists work within different health systems and different cultures, have different roles and responsibilities and apply different skills, which cannot be elucidated systematically in a survey. Although psychiatrists consider themselves as carrying a well-defined identity determined by commonalities in values and skills and shared memberships of professional organizations, they also possess many unquantifiable differences. This applies even more so to less precisely defined categories such as nurses and psychologists.

Some categories are even more fluid. An example is community services, despite careful definitions that were discussed and agreed in advance in principle. However, concepts such as community or user involvement can have very different meanings or interpretations across the Region in practice, related to cultural, political and health system tradition and development. A community-based psychiatric inpatient unit in one country can be an institution in another. Perceived involvement of service users in one country is oppression in another. This report has attempted to clarify such conceptual variability by presenting examples from a range of countries.

The European Region is still diverse, but evidence emerging from this baseline survey shows that mental health policies, interventions and services show a trend towards convergence. Most policies and legislations cover a comparable scope. Most countries now provide some community services, although in some on a small pilot scale and supported by international nongovernmental organizations. The involvement of service users and carers is mostly accepted as good practice, although implementation differs. It is to be hoped that this convergence will progress, eventually offering the comprehensive range of mental health activities stated by the priorities of the Mental Health Declaration for Europe:

i. foster awareness of the importance of mental well-being;
ii. collectively tackle stigma, discrimination and inequality, and empower and support people with mental health problems and their families to be actively engaged in this process;
iii. design and implement comprehensive, integrated and efficient mental health systems that cover promotion, prevention, treatment and rehabilitation, care and recovery;
iv. address the need for a competent workforce, effective in all these areas; and
v. recognize the experience and knowledge of service users and carers as an important basis for planning and developing mental health services.

The discussion at the end of each chapter has already raised many of the challenges and priorities for further action. More specifically, it is important to judge the data in this report against the 12 milestones in the Mental Health Action Plan for Europe. These were agreed with Member States who committed themselves to move towards these milestones by 2010. This survey indicates progress on each of the milestones.

1. Prepare policies and implement activities to counter stigma and discrimination and promote mental well-being, including in healthy schools and workplaces

Almost 80% of countries have carried out activities to tackle stigma and discrimination, although fewer countries in south-eastern Europe and CIS countries. Government agencies are involved in most countries, especially as funders, but nongovernmental organizations and, to a lesser extent, professional associations often play an active role in delivery. Programmes targeting the mental health of students in school settings are inconsistently implemented, although most countries have mental health specialists available in schools. Few countries have developed programmes that systematically address mental health in the workplace. Related to this, several countries have developed policies to prevent stress in the workplace in partnership between the employment and health sectors.

These data do not inform about local initiatives, and many schools and workplaces may well have initiated excellent practices, irrespective of national policies. If so, they have not been disseminated effectively.

Striking was the lack of evaluation of programmes covered by this milestone, despite the investment. This is likely to hinder the adoption of such programmes elsewhere. Two recent joint publications by Health Scotland and the WHO Regional Office for Europe[1] describe a good example of a systematic and comprehensive approach to developing, implementing and evaluating an anti-stigma campaign.

2. Scrutinize the mental health impact of public policy

Just over one third of countries perform a health impact assessment, mostly in the form of population mental health surveys or service accreditation. Mental health impact assessment of policy – systematic evaluation of the effects of implementing policy on the mental health of the population or vulnerable groups – was not mentioned. This subject has raised interest, and some initiatives have taken place under recent EU presidencies. More wide-ranging attempts need to be undertaken, technology developed and results disseminated.

1 Stigma: an international briefing paper. Edinburgh, Health Scotland, 2008 (http://www.healthscotland.com/uploads/documents/6421-Stigma_Guidebook_for_Action%202635.pdf, accessed 8 May 2008). Stigma: a guidebook for action. Edinburgh, Health Scotland, 2008 (http://www.healthscotland.com/uploads/documents/6422-Stigma_An_International_Briefing_Paper_2704.pdf, accessed 8 May 2008).

3. Include the prevention of mental health problems and suicide in national policies

About one quarter of countries introduced policies or programmes to prevent suicide by reducing access to lethal means or by recognizing and treating at-risk population groups in primary health or specialized care settings during the past five years. In some groups of countries, the number of countries that have policies is higher than the number that had implemented programmes. This is either due to a lag period of implementation or because some countries have wide-ranging policies that are beyond the scope of implementation. In contrast, some EU15 countries had programmes but not policies.

Especially many EU15 and other high-income countries have introduced policies and programmes that aim to prevent depression, targeting the whole population. Far fewer countries have developed and implemented programmes targeting vulnerable groups, such as the children of parents with mental health problems, women (postpartum depression), employees or bereaved widows and widowers. Considering the greater effectiveness and efficiency of targeted programmes, this is an area for potential development.

4. Develop specialist services capable of addressing the specific challenges of the young and older people, and gender specific issues

Young people are mostly reasonably well addressed in stigma and well-being campaigns. In contrast, few countries reach out to older people. Fewer specialist services are generally available for older people as compared with children and adolescents. The exception is residential facilities. These have very different functions for these two groups and cannot therefore meaningfully be compared. More countries offer specialist training to psychiatrists for treating children than for psychiatrists for older people. The impression is of bias against old people.

Quite consistently, more women attended outpatient clinics, whereas admission to hospitals was more balanced, with a bias towards men. There are many possible explanations, including women more often targeted or more receptive to prevention activities and asking for help at an earlier stage.

Few countries could offer information on the number and distribution of beds and places by sex. The explanation for this was the need for flexibility, allowing mixed occupancy as required. This raises the question of whether wards are mixed in some countries and how this is managed to create a safe and dignified environment, especially for women.

5. Prioritize services that target the mental health problems of marginalized and vulnerable groups, including problems of comorbidity, i.e. where mental health problems occur jointly with other problems such as substance misuse or physical illness

About two thirds of countries have developed policies or programmes to prevent mental health problems among vulnerable groups. The target groups vary considerably, from the Roma population in south-eastern Europe to minorities and refugees in many countries in western Europe.

A specific challenge for ethnic and minority groups is access to services. This is very inconsistent, if known at all, with 25% of countries reporting underrepresentation and equal representation. Very few countries report overrepresentation. This has to be interpreted in the light of very different combinations and characteristics of minority groups across countries, and this is an important subject for further analysis.

A concern is the neglect of physical health care offered to people diagnosed with a mental disorder. There are numerous formal arrangements between mental health services and other health agencies covering primary care, HIV and AIDS, reproductive health, adolescent health and substance misuse disorders. It would be valuable to have data on the number of cross-referrals, treatment offered and particularly the experience of service users.

6. Develop partnership for intersectoral working and address disincentives that hinder joint working

Formal collaborative agreements often exist between the mental health sector and education, welfare, services for older people and the criminal justice system, especially in the EU. There are some relative gaps, such as the lack of partnerships with employment and housing in some countries. It is not known how effectively these formal partnerships operate in practice, particularly under pressure.

Some of the initiatives are local and small scale, especially in the eastern part of the Region, where nongovernmental organizations fund and deliver many activities. This raises questions about sustainability and diffusion. There is a great difference between some of the universal programmes in EU15 countries and the local pilot programmes in other countries. Few evaluations of such pilot services are available. Comparative work is necessary to determine whether some of the large-scale programmes in high-income countries in Europe could be efficient in less affluent countries.

7. Introduce human resource strategies to build up a sufficient and competent mental health workforce

Fewer than half the countries have a national workforce strategy. The variation in numbers, skill mix and training of the workforce is considerable, even within countries, raising questions about quality across the Region and consistency in treatment and care practices.

Continuing education lacks regulation; it is often informal and provided by external agencies, sometimes with a conflict of interest. A few countries have introduced regulation and guidance that could form a model of good practice, possibly in partnership with international agencies committed to this field such as the European Union of Medical Specialists.

Remarkably few countries could provide information about the number of psychiatrists and nurses immigrating or emigrating. Since this is a source of major concern for workforce planning, particularly in lower-income countries, this is issue needs attention.

8. Define a set of indicators on the determinants and epidemiology of mental health and for the design and delivery of services in partnership with other Member States

All countries collect a minimum data set covering hospital information data. Data on community mental health and especially social care activities are less often available. In many countries, such data sets are probably not collected, and some countries are still in the process of developing software. There are no known examples of different countries using identical or compatible software on a national scale.

Attempts have been made repeatedly to agree on indicators, particularly across the EU. Some basic indicators are available, predictably mostly related to hospital activities. Although it is easily agreed that indicators need to be specific, measurable, achievable, realistic and timely (SMART), their development is quite challenging for a dynamic area such as mental health. The lack of precise responses from many countries to a proportion of the questions in this survey, agreed and tested in advance, shows the challenge ahead. Nevertheless, this priority cannot be avoided if countries intend to manage their reform and desire to benefit from advances elsewhere.

9. Confirm health funding, regulation and legislation that is equitable and inclusive of mental health

Investment in mental health is generally higher as a proportion of the health budget in higher-income countries than lower-income countries, with implications for service development, quality of care and equity. The proportion of spending on mental health promotion and mental disorder prevention is always very low, probably absent in some of the lowest-income countries, with implications for inclusiveness and fairness.

Medication should be freely available for vulnerable people, at least in principle. In the lowest-income countries, supply is not always sufficient, and families and service users may end up paying out of pocket. Psychosocial therapy more often relies on co-payments. Since some forms of brief psychological interventions are as effective and cost the same as medication, with fewer unwanted side effects, shifting investment might be worth considering.

Distribution of funding should favour the most vulnerable and poorest population groups. Few countries distribute funding based on an equitable formula. A comparison of techniques and formulas used across the Region might be instructive.

10. End inhumane and degrading treatment and care and enact human rights and mental health legislation to comply with the standards of United Nations conventions and international legislation

Most countries have modern policies and legislation, many developed since the Mental Health Declaration for Europe was endorsed, incorporating many of the priorities and actions of the Declaration. It is less clear whether these countries have implemented these policies and legislation. This report describes some instances of the implementation of good practice without the presence of policy. The role of primary care in diagnosing and treating people with common and severe mental health problems is an example.

The development of community-based services in many countries has increased choice and access to a range of services, as detailed in this report. The reliance on mental hospitals is still high in parts of the Region but declining gradually. The gap between policy and practice in the coverage of some essential components of community-based services such as 24-hour crisis care needs to be addressed with some urgency.

Nevertheless, some countries have given examples of degrading practices that are still in existence, particularly related to institutions such as mental hospitals and social care homes. These countries express their commitment to change but are struggling due to a combination of infrastructure limitations, economic pressure, workforce shortages and cultural factors. Changing conditions and care practices in these places is one of the highest priorities for the next few years, which will require the solidarity of other countries in the WHO European Region.

Information needs to be collected on safeguarding the human rights of people with mental disorders, such as reviewing procedures to prevent poor practices and abuse related to involuntary admission and treatment and the effectiveness of alternatives to restraint or seclusion.

Despite the legal right to legal representation free of charge in almost all countries, access and affordability of legal representation is very poor in some countries. Without such representation, service users are unlikely to be in a position to enforce their rights, and this needs attention.

11. Increase the level of social inclusion of people with mental health problems

Mental health problems are the major cause of disability in many countries. People with mental health problems have lower workforce participation than that of people with other health problems. Most countries recognize the challenge this poses and have introduced disability legislation that includes disability due to mental health problems.

Most countries have legislation that guarantees financial support for housing or incentives to employ people with disability, particularly in the EU. These entitlements are generic: addressing the group of people with disability as a whole, and not always enforced, and people with mental health problems can be selectively excluded from employment opportunities. Further information on equitable access for people with mental health problems is important.

12. Ensure representation of users and carers on committees and groups responsible for the planning, delivery, review and inspection of mental health activities

There has been considerable progress in the recognition of service users and carers as partners on bodies that are responsible for planning, running and monitoring mental health activities, although mainly in EU15 countries. This is one of the areas with the sharpest gradation across the Region. Involvement of service users is strongly associated with the involvement of carers and government support.

Representation of service users and carers on inspection visits to mental facilities, a commitment in the Mental Health Declaration for Europe, is far from standard in every part of the Region. A differentiation also needs to be made between acting as a full member of a statutory review team and being included on a visit of a foreign nongovernmental organization, without any status. The recognition that the involvement of service users and carers is good practice is a hopeful sign of future progress. This is an area where lessons can be learned from the experiences of the countries that have introduced such practices.

WHO action

The conclusions of this report indicate the need for future activities the WHO Regional Office for Europe needs to pursue on behalf of its Member States and as mandated in the Mental Health Declaration for Europe. To meet the challenges and opportunities identified in this survey, the WHO Regional Office for Europe will:

(a) Partnership
  i. encourage cooperation in this area with intergovernmental organizations, including the European Commission and the Council of Europe;

(b) Health information
  i. support Member States in developing mental health surveillance;
  ii. produce comparative data on the state and progress of mental health and mental health services in Member States;

(c) Research
  i. establish a network of mental health collaborating centres that offer opportunities for international partnerships, high-quality research and the exchange of researchers;
  ii. produce and disseminate the best available evidence on good practice, taking into account the ethical aspects of mental health;

(d) Policy and service development
  i. support governments by providing expertise to underpin mental health reform through effective mental health policies that include legislation, service design, promoting mental health and preventing mental health problems;
  ii. offer assistance in setting up train-the-trainer programmes;
  iii. initiate exchange schemes for innovators;
  iv. assist in formulating research policies and questions;
  v. encourage change agents by setting up a network of national leaders of reform and key civil servants;

(e) Advocacy
  i. inform and monitor policies and activities that will promote the human rights and inclusion of people with mental health problems and reduce stigma and discrimination against them;

ii. empower the users of mental health services, carers and nongovernmental organizations with information and coordinate activities across countries;
iii. support Member States in developing an information base to help empower the users of mental health services;
iv. facilitate international exchanges of experience by key regional and local nongovernmental organizations; and
v. provide the mass media, nongovernmental organizations and other interested groups and individuals with objective and constructive information.

In summary, this report co-funded by the European Commission shows that countries in the WHO European Region are committed to transforming their mental health programmes and activities, aiming to shift from institutional practices to person-centred community-based care. The very large majority of countries have made significant progress over the past few years, and several are among the leaders in the world in such areas as mental health promotion, mental disorder prevention activities, service reform and human rights. However, this report also identifies weaknesses in Europe, some systematically so, such as the lack of consensus on definitions and the absence of compatible data collection, and others that show a high degree of variation, such as the need for development and investment in several areas. We anticipate that the next few years will see further progress towards the vision and the milestones of the Mental Health Declaration for Europe. WHO is committed to assist this process.

Annexes

Annex 1. Contributors from countries

Albania:	Neli Demi, Ledia Lazeri
Austria:	Barbara Weibold, Heinz Katschnig
Azerbaijan:	Sevil Asadova
Belgium:	Pol Gerits, Jan Van de Velde
Bosnia and Herzegovina	
Federation of Bosnia and Herzegovina:	Vesna Puratic, Goran Cerkez, Taida Kapetanovic
Republika Srpska:	Biljana Lakic, Milan Latinovic, Natalija Milovanovic
Bulgaria:	Hristo Hinkov, Angel Broshtilov, Zahari Zarkov, Michail Okoliyski
Croatia:	Neven Henigsberg, Elizabeta Radonic
Cyprus:	Costas Kyranides, Evangelos Anastasiou
Czech Republic:	Cyril Hoschl , Barbora Wenigova, Eva Dragomericka
Denmark:	Marianne Jespersen
Estonia:	Airi Värnik, Merike Sisask, Kaire Adamsoo, Andres Lehtmets
Finland:	Kristian Wahlbeck, Eija Stengård
France:	Ministry of Health
Georgia:	Manana Sharashidze, Akaki Gamkrelidze, Nana Zavradashvili, Giorgi Khufenia
Germany:	Aktion Psychisch Kranke e.V.
Greece:	Pavlos Theodorakis, the Department of Mental Health of the Greek Ministry of Health and Social Solidarity and the Mental Health Programme Support Unit.
Hungary:	Istvan Bitter, Kinga Szepeshazi
Ireland:	Ciara Pidgeon, Cliodhna Daly
Israel:	Alona Baidani-Auerbach, Inna Pugachova
Italy:	Teresa di Fiandra, Andrea Gaddini, Giuseppe Tibaldi, Floriana Lo Bianco
Latvia:	Maris Taube
Lithuania:	Ona Davidoniene, Jelena Stanislavoviene
Luxembourg:	Charles B. Pull
Malta:	Ray G. Xerri
Moldova:	Larisa Boderscova, Anatol Nacu, Pavel Ursu, Mihai Ciocanu
Montenegro:	Zorica Barac-Otasevic, Tatijana Mandic, Miodrag Radunovic
Netherlands:	Marijke Ruiter, Jan Walburg
Norway:	Freja Ulvestad Kärki
Poland:	Czesław Czabała, Grazyna Herczynska
Portugal:	Antonio Leuschner, Miguel Xavier
Romania:	Dan Ghenea, Bogdana Tudorache, Domnica Petrovai
Russian Federation:	Zurab I. Kekelidze, Olga Leonova
Serbia:	Dusica Lecic Tosevski, Milica Pejovic Milovancevic, Aleksandra Milicevic Kalasic
Slovakia:	Eva Palova
Slovenia:	Andrej Marusic, Nadja Cobal
Spain	Manuel Gomez-Beneyto
Castilla y León:	José Manuel Martínez Rodríguez
Catalonia:	Cristina Molina
Extremadura:	Miguel Simón
Galicia:	Fernando Márquez
Murcia:	Carlos Giribert
Sweden:	Helena Silfverhielm, Claes-Göran Stefansson
Switzerland:	Regula Ricka, Franz Wyss, Paul Camenzind, Herbert Heise
The former Yugoslav Republic of Macedonia:	Snezana Cicevalieva, Antoni Novotni, Stojan Bajraktarov
Turkey:	Bilal Aytac, Saime Sahinöz
United Kingdom	
England and Wales:	Susannah Howard, Louis Appleby, Anita Wadhawan, Simon Pearson
Scotland:	Scottish Government Health Directorates
Uzbekistan:	Nargiza Khodjaeva

Annex 2. Mental Health Declaration for Europe

Facing the Challenges, Building Solutions

WHO European Ministerial Conference on Mental Health
Helsinki, Finland 12-15 January 2005

Preamble

1. We, the Ministers of Health of Member States in the European Region of the World Health Organization (WHO), in the presence of the European Commissioner for Health and Consumer Protection, together with the WHO Regional Director for Europe, meeting at the WHO Ministerial Conference on Mental Health, held in Helsinki from 12 to 15 January 2005, acknowledge that mental health and mental well-being are fundamental to the quality of life and productivity of individuals, families, communities and nations, enabling people to experience life as meaningful and to be creative and active citizens. We believe that the primary aim of mental health activity is to enhance people's well-being and functioning by focusing on their strengths and resources, reinforcing resilience and enhancing protective external factors.

2. We recognize that the promotion of mental health and the prevention, treatment, care and rehabilitation of mental health problems are a priority for WHO and its Member States, the European Union (EU) and the Council of Europe, as expressed in resolutions by the World Health Assembly and the WHO Executive Board, the WHO Regional Committee for Europe and the Council of the European Union. These resolutions urge Member States, WHO, the EU and the Council of Europe to take action to relieve the burden of mental health problems and to improve mental well-being.

3. We recall our commitment to resolution EUR/RC51/R5 on the Athens Declaration on Mental Health, Man-made Disasters, Stigma and Community Care and to resolution EUR/RC53/R4 adopted by the WHO Regional Committee for Europe in September 2003, expressing concern that the disease burden from mental disorders in Europe is not diminishing and that many people with mental health problems do not receive the treatment and care they need, despite the development of effective interventions. The Regional Committee requested the Regional Director to:
   - give high priority to mental health issues when implementing activities concerning the update of the Health for All policy;
   - arrange a ministerial conference on mental health in Europe in Helsinki in January 2005.

4. We note resolutions that support an action programme on mental health. Resolution EB109.R8, adopted by the WHO Executive Board in January 2002, supported by World Health Assembly resolution WHA55.10 in May 2002, calls on WHO Member States to:
   - adopt the recommendations contained in The world health report 2001;
   - establish mental health policies, programmes and legislation based on current knowledge and considerations regarding human rights, in consultation with all stakeholders in mental health;
   - increase investment in mental health, both within countries and in bilateral and multilateral cooperation, as an integral component of the well-being of populations.

5. Resolutions of the Council of the European Union, recommendations of the Council of Europe and WHO resolutions dating back to 1975 recognize the important role of mental health promotion and the damaging association between mental health problems and social marginalization, unemployment, homelessness and alcohol and other substance use disorders. We accept the importance of the provisions of the Convention for the Protection of Human Rights and Fundamental Freedoms, of the Convention on the Rights of the Child, of the European Convention for the Prevention of Torture and Inhuman or Degrading Treatment or Punishment and of the European Social Charter, as well as the Council of Europe's commitment to the protection and promotion of mental health which has been developed through the Declaration of its Ministerial Conference on Mental Health in the Future (Stockholm, 1985) and through its other recommendations adopted in this field, in particular Recommendation R(90)22 on protection of the mental health of certain vulnerable groups in society and Recommendation Rec(2004)10 concerning the protection of the human rights and dignity of persons with mental disorder.

Scope

6. We note that many aspects of mental health policy and services are experiencing a transformation across the European Region. Policy and services are striving to achieve social inclusion and equity, taking a comprehensive view of the balance between the needs and benefits of diverse mental health activities aimed at the population as a whole, groups at risk and people with mental health problems. Services are being provided in a wide range of community-based settings and no longer exclusively in isolated and large institutions. We believe that this is the right and necessary direction. We welcome the fact that policy and practice on mental health now cover:
   - I. the promotion of mental well-being;
   - II. the tackling of stigma, discrimination and social exclusion;
   - III. the prevention of mental health problems;
   - IV. care for people with mental health problems, providing comprehensive and effective services and interventions, offering service users and carers[1] involvement and choice;
   - V. the recovery and inclusion into society of those who have experienced serious mental health problems.

Priorities

7 We need to build on the platform of reform and modernization in the WHO European Region, learn from our shared experiences and be aware of the unique characteristics of individual countries. We believe that the main priorities for the next decade are to:
   - I. foster awareness of the importance of mental well-being;
   - II. collectively tackle stigma, discrimination and inequality, and empower and support people with mental health problems and their families to be actively engaged in this process;
   - III. design and implement comprehensive, integrated and efficient mental health systems that cover promotion, prevention, treatment and rehabilitation, care and recovery;
   - IV. address the need for a competent workforce, effective in all these areas;
   - V. recognize the experience and knowledge of service users and carers as an important basis for planning and developing mental health services.

Actions

8. We endorse the statement that there is no health without mental health. Mental health is central to the human, social and economic capital of nations and should therefore be considered as an integral and essential part of other public policy areas such as human rights, social care, education and employment. Therefore we, ministers responsible for health, commit ourselves, subject to national constitutional structures and responsibilities, to recognizing the need for comprehensive evidence-based mental health policies and to considering ways and means of developing, implementing and reinforcing such policies in our countries. These policies, aimed at achieving mental well-being and social inclusion of people with mental health problems, require actions in the following areas:
   - I. promote the mental well-being of the population as a whole by measures that aim to create awareness and positive change for individuals and families, communities and civil society, educational and working environments, and governments and national agencies;
   - II. consider the potential impact of all public policies on mental health, with particular attention to vulnerable groups, demonstrating the centrality of mental health in building a healthy, inclusive and productive society;
   - III. tackle stigma and discrimination, ensure the protection of human rights and dignity and implement the necessary legislation in order to empower people at risk or suffering from mental health problems and disabilities to participate fully and equally in society;
   - IV. offer targeted support and interventions sensitive to the life stages of people at risk, particularly the parenting and education of children and young people and the care of older people;

---

1 The term "carer" is used here to describe a family member, friend or other informal care-giver.

V. develop and implement measures to reduce the preventable causes of mental health problems, comorbidity and suicide;
VI. build up the capacity and ability of general practitioners and primary care services, networking with specialized medical and non-medical care, to offer effective access, identification and treatments to people with mental health problems;
VII. offer people with severe mental health problems effective and comprehensive care and treatment in a range of settings and in a manner which respects their personal preferences and protects them from neglect and abuse;
VIII. establish partnership, coordination and leadership across regions, countries, sectors and agencies that have an influence on the mental health and social inclusion of individuals and families, groups and communities;
IX. design recruitment and education and training programmes to create a sufficient and competent multidisciplinary workforce;
X. assess the mental health status and needs of the population, specific groups and individuals in a manner that allows comparison nationally and internationally;
XI. provide fair and adequate financial resources to deliver these aims;
XII. initiate research and support evaluation and dissemination of the above actions.

9. We recognize the importance and the urgency of facing the challenges and building solutions based on evidence. We therefore endorse the Mental Health Action Plan for Europe and support its implementation across the WHO European Region, each country adapting the points appropriate to its needs and resources. We are also committed to showing solidarity across the Region and to sharing knowledge, best practice and expertise.

Responsibilities

10. We, the Ministers of Health of the Member States in the WHO European Region, commit ourselves to supporting the implementation of the following measures, in accordance with each country's constitutional structures and policies and national and subnational needs, circumstances and resources:

I. enforce mental health policy and legislation that sets standards for mental health activities and upholds human rights;
II. coordinate responsibility for the formulation, dissemination and implementation of policies and legislation relevant to mental health within government;
III. assess the public mental health impact of government action;
IV. eliminate stigma and discrimination and enhance inclusion by increasing public awareness and empowering people at risk;
V. offer people with mental health problems choice and involvement in their own care, sensitive to their needs and culture;
VI. review and if necessary introduce equal opportunity or anti-discrimination legislation;
VII. promote mental health in education and employment, communities and other relevant settings by increasing collaboration between agencies responsible for health and other relevant sectors;
VIII. prevent risk factors where they occur, for instance, by supporting the development of working environments conducive to mental health and creating incentives for the provision of support at work or the earliest return for those who have recovered from mental health problems;
IX. address suicide prevention and the causes of harmful stress, violence, depression, anxiety and alcohol and other substance use disorders;
X. recognize and enhance the central role of primary health care and general practitioners and strengthen their capacity to take on responsibility for mental health;
XI. develop community-based services to replace care in large institutions for those with severe mental health problems;
XII. enforce measure that end inhumane and degrading care;
XIII. enhance partnerships between agencies responsible for care and support such as health, benefits, housing, education and employment;

XIV. include mental health in the curricula of all health professionals and design continuous professional education and training programmes for the mental health workforce;
XV. encourage the development of specialized expertise within the mental health workforce, to address the specific needs of groups such as children, young people, older people and those with long-term and severe mental health problems;
XVI. provide sufficient resources for mental health, considering the burden of disease, and make investment in mental health an identifiable part of overall health expenditure, in order to achieve parity with investments in other areas of health;
XVII. develop surveillance of positive mental well-being and mental health problems, including risk factors and help-seeking behaviour, and monitor implementation;
XVIII. commission research when and where knowledge or technology is insufficient and disseminate findings.

11. We will support nongovernmental organizations active in the mental health field and stimulate the creation of nongovernmental and service user organizations. We particularly welcome organizations active in:
I. organizing users who are engaged in developing their own activities, including the setting up and running of self-help groups and training in recovery competencies;
II. empowering vulnerable and marginalized people and advocating their case;
III. providing community-based services involving users;
IV. developing the caring and coping skills and competencies of families and carers, and their active involvement in care programmes;
V. setting up schemes to improve parenting, education and tolerance and to tackle alcohol and other substance use disorders, violence and crime;
VI. developing local services that target the needs of marginalized groups;
VII. running help lines and internet counselling for people in crisis situations, suffering from violence or at risk of suicide;
VIII. creating employment opportunities for disabled people.

12. We call upon the European Commission and the Council of Europe to support the implementation of this WHO Mental Health Declaration for Europe on the basis of their respective competences.

13. We request the Regional Director of WHO Europe to take action in the following areas:
(a) **Partnership**
I. encourage cooperation in this area with intergovernmental organizations, including the European Commission and the Council of Europe.

(b) **Health information**
I. support Member States in the development of mental health surveillance;
II. produce comparative data on the state and progress of mental health and mental health services in Member States.

(c) **Research**
I. establish a network of mental health collaborating centres that offer opportunities for international partnerships, good quality research and the exchange of researchers;
II. produce and disseminate the best available evidence on good practice, taking into account the ethical aspects of mental health.

(d) **Policy and service development**
I. support governments by providing expertise to underpin mental health reform through effective mental health policies that include legislation, service design, promotion of mental health and prevention of mental health problems;

II. offer assistance with setting up "train the trainer" programmes;
III. initiate exchange schemes for innovators;
IV. assist with the formulation of research policies and questions;
V. encourage change agents by setting up a network of national leaders of reform and key civil servants.

(e) **Advocacy**

I. inform and monitor policies and activities that will promote the human rights and inclusion of people with mental health problems and reduce stigma and discrimination against them;
II. empower users, carers and nongovernmental organizations with information and coordinate activities across countries;
III. support Member States in developing an information base to help empower the users of mental health services;
IV. facilitate international exchanges of experience by key regional and local nongovernmental organizations;
V. provide the media, nongovernmental organizations and other interested groups and individuals with objective and constructive information.

14. We request the WHO Regional Office for Europe to take the necessary steps to ensure that mental health policy development and implementation are fully supported and that adequate priority and resources are given to activities and programmes to fulfil the requirements of this Declaration.

15. We commit ourselves to reporting back to WHO on the progress of implementation of this Declaration in our countries at an intergovernmental meeting to be held before 2010.

Minister of Health and Social Services of Finland

WHO Regional Director for Europe